GASTROPARESIS:

A ROADMAP FOR YOUR JOURNEY

Chelsey M McIntyre, PharmD

Gastroparesis: A Roadmap for Your Journey

Copyright © 2017 by Chelsey McIntyre.

This book contains advice and information relating to health care. It should be used to supplement rather than replace the advice of your doctor and other trained health professionals. All efforts have been made to assure the accuracy of the information contained in this book as of the date of publication.

FIRST EDITION

ISBN (Paperback): 978-0-9986761-0-4
ISBN (eBook): 978-0-9986761-1-1

For each person who had a reason to open this book. Yours is a journey worth navigating.

Contents

Part I

Introduction 1

"*Each patient carries his own doctor inside of him. They come to us not knowing the truth. We are at our best when we give the doctor that resides within each patient a chance to go to work.*"

ALBERT SCHWEITZER

The concept for this book has been bouncing around my brain for years. To be honest, I never felt that I was ready to write it, or that I had enough to offer to make it worthwhile. However, as I explained my condition to a new acquaintance, I suddenly realized that my experience with gastroparesis and my clinical training had morphed into a unique understanding and perspective on the condition.

I knew that the me of years past, with all of the confusion and disorientation I felt for many years after my diagnosis, would have given quite a bit to know what I know now. And I had to share that knowledge in the hopes that it could be of use to someone else in a similar situation. This mix of experience and knowledge regarding gastroparesis and health come from the following:

- Fourteen years of living with severe gastroparesis
- A Doctor of Pharmacy degree
- Clinical pharmacy residency training
- Six years of practice as a clinical pharmacist

My intent in this book is not to prescribe a lifestyle, treatment, or outlook. My goal is to provide the tools necessary for every person to better understand how to navigate this condition, along with sound medical information and advice stemming from my professional and personal experiences. I have no disclosures regarding personal or financial relationships nor any incentive for personal gain from the topics to be discussed.

Most information found here will be interpreted differently for each person and each situation. All recommendations, advice, or ideas related to medical treatment should always be discussed with a medical provider familiar with your situation.

HOW TO USE THIS BOOK

This book was written with the objective of helping you to become an empowered self-advocate. This involves having the knowledge and confidence to interpret and understand your options, ask the right questions, and be fully involved in your own care and health status.

You'll notice that the book has a somewhat unique format with a large margin on each page that contains information of its own. This was done to improve readability and focus within the text, moving all other notes and points to a separate location. Everything that can be found in the margin correlates directly to the text that is right alongside it. This will include images and visual representations of what is being discussed, side notes and comments, and bottom-line summaries for complicated topics. These same margins can be used by you for your personal notes on the information that is being covered and how it applies directly to your journey and experiences.

Here is where you will find side notes or even summaries on the topics being discussed in the main text.

The rest of this open space can be used by you!

The information in the book is meant to build on itself. The first chapter will provide information that will make the second chapter easier to understand, and so on. Any time a topic which was already discussed is mentioned again, the page number is referenced for easy review. There is also an index available in the back of the book to allow for quick navigation to specific topics. However, the most value will be gained by reading the book all the way through before hopping around.

The first and largest section of this book provides general and foundational information. This will weave together to provide you with a thorough understanding for the GI tract, how medications work, the implications of gastroparesis and related GI conditions, and many of the terms that are often thrown around. It will also teach you how to evaluate and interpret the information that you find when doing your own research and when new ideas or treatments are suggested to you by friends, family members, or doctors. The goal is for you to walk away from this section armed with the ability to face the questions, doubts, fears, and uncertainties that gastroparesis can present.

Here is where you might find a summary of the information being discussed in the text, such as:

Part 1: Provides foundational information that will help you in making decisions throughout the future

Part 2: Provides focused information on specific medical topics and treatments

The second section of this book addresses specific questions and issues that stem from having gastroparesis and many of its complications. This includes the medications and treatments that are often used with gastroparesis and related GI conditions, as well as notes to consider for medications that are used to treat other conditions. While the first section is meant to empower you on the topics of gastroparesis and health as a whole, the second section is meant to provide sound information regarding specific medical concerns that commonly arise for those of us with gastroparesis.

You will also find that my personal experience with gastroparesis is sprinkled throughout the book. Learning about the experiences of others has always been helpful to me in a variety of ways, from emotional reassurance to shaping my own management plan. I made every effort to be sincere and genuine in the recounting of my journey, and I hope that this may, in turn, be helpful to others.

Study Participation
Fill out a 1-2 minute survey now, and then one more time when you finish the book. The study will be used in a larger effort to make such services readily available through doctor's offices and paid for via health insurance.

In order to evaluate how this type of guidance can improve quality of life for people with gastroparesis (and chronic diagnoses in general), I have created an opportunity for you to participate in a voluntary study. See the margin for the details!

www.yourgijourney.com/s1

Personal Experience Part 1

One week of a bad flu hit me pretty hard at the age of 17. It was April of my senior year of high school and I was out for a few days with my head over the toilet. Eventually it ran its course, and I got back to my typical daily life. But one thing wasn't quite right – I still seemed to be throwing up my food.

I had just recovered from an infection that caused me to throw up everything that I ate, so continuing to throw up didn't seem that odd until it continued for a couple of weeks after the flu had clearly ended. I wasn't quite nauseated, and my muscles weren't achy, but for some reason, many of the things that I ate seemed to end up back in my mouth and then the toilet. When I realized that the food I had eaten for an early dinner the night before was coming up in the morning after I woke, I really started to get worried.

Over the final month of my senior year, I began to expect to have food regurgitate into my mouth at all times of the day, and feel food sitting in my belly for hours on end. This was already uncomfortable, but then I started to bring up the water that I habitually drank, increasing my discomfort further. At the time, I had a very healthy diet consisting primarily of fresh salads and sandwiches and multiple liters of water a day. To my dismay, the water that I drank was suddenly shooting up my throat and into my mouth with force, making it difficult for me to keep it from coming out. At a college course that I took that first summer, the water actually came out of my mouth while I was sitting in class and landed on the desk. That mortifying experience quickly ended my habit of drinking water in public and dramatically reduced the amount of water that I drank at all.

After a few months, it became clear that whatever was wrong with me was not going to go away on its own. I was in pain, bloated, and gassy consistently, and there always seemed to be food in my mouth. I had, of course, tried to Google everything but had come up empty. Did I do this to myself somehow, or was I really sick? If I was really sick, how bad was it?

I finally got a referral to see a gastrointestinal (GI) doctor about these issues. He ordered a barium swallow. For those that have not had one of those, it is exactly what it sounds like. I swallowed a lot of barium and they looked at how it traveled through my esophagus and stomach. The technician performing the test suddenly chastised me for eating break-fast that morning even though I was supposed to fast. "What?" I said, "I haven't eaten since I had dinner around 7 last night." To my surprise, he laughed at me and told me that I was wasting my time lying to him. Although I had a very quiet and shy demeanor at the time, I raised my voice and insisted that I had not eaten, and I wanted to know why he did not believe me.

The test results came back the next week: "No apparent anomalies of upper GI tract upon barium swallow except for food in the stomach. Patient claims to not have eaten since previous evening."

While the technician had no idea what he was looking at, this must have clued my GI doctor into thinking that I was having issues with proper stomach emptying. He told me that I was "like a cow chewing cud" and that I should appreciate the humor. I didn't. He then prescribed Reglan (metoclopramide) and told me to take it 3 times a day, before each meal, and let him know if I still had symptoms.

A week later, I experienced an extreme spasm in my neck while I was driving and almost crashed my car into the concrete median. The next day I had a similar spasm in my thigh while walking to a class. It sud-denly occurred to me that I should check and see what the side effects were to this supposedly safe medication that the doctor had prescribed. And there it was – spasms. It didn't help that right next to that were some other, really frightening sounding, side effects, such as something called tardive dyskinesia. It was merely a quick Google search, but I was pretty certain I had figured out what was causing this new, dangerous problem.

I called my doctor to inform him of my concerns and, after waiting three days for a response, he simply stated "Oh yeah, that happens with that medication. I will refer you to another GI doctor that might have more experience with your situation. Until then, you should keep taking the Reglan." Needless to say, I did not keep taking the Reglan. In retrospect, I should have told the physician that I was planning to stop, but was too intimidated to speak up.

2 Finding Information

Most people with a gastroparesis diagnosis know that their doctors are not very good at giving any guidance on what to do with the diagnosis. In fact, some aren't even very good at explaining what, exactly, gastroparesis is. I know that one of the things that I did at the most crucial points in time – when I first had symptoms, first started taking medications, first received my diagnosis - was Google everything. I wanted to know the WHY of everything. I have been told by many people that I am an overly curious person in general, but I know that everyone I have spoken to with gastroparesis has also felt left to dig up explanations and information for themselves.

The internet is a wealth of information. It is right at our fingertips and it is there to provide at least some form of an answer to almost any question we could ever ask. I have learned uncountable things from the internet, not the least of which was what gastroparesis is and that Reglan could cause severe and sometimes permanent spasms. The internet can help anyone become more informed, but only when using the right resources.

Some recent reviews of medical information on the internet have yielded some very concerning results. For instance, when attempting to answer over 250 different medical questions, one review found that the sites which most often show up at the top of the search results, including Wikipedia and Medscape, answered 12–21% of those questions wrong. Another review found that RxList.com, a website that people often use to find information about their medications, answered 35% of questions incorrectly. Those are frightening rates for finding bad information, particularly when they concern something as valuable as our health.

Many sites have popped up these past few years claiming to help with all types of chronic conditions, including gastroparesis and other functional GI disorders. Unfortunately, most of the information on these websites is not based on evidence. This can mean a number of things, including that the information or advice has not actually been shown to work and much of it is not even based off of scientifically reasonable assumptions – when looked at from the perspective of how the disease works, the treatment does not make any logical sense.

In addition, some of these suggestions and ideas may actually be dangerous. The dangers could include preventing adequate nutrition, suggesting not thinking for yourself or listening to your own concerns, or by actually being harmful to your body and your health. There are an unfortunate number of people out there that are interested in making money off of their suggestions. Some of these people may have good intentions; some of them may believe that they are doing no harm. But when the suggestions are not based on evidence, the results could be very bad.

A key rule to follow: Just because you read it or heard about it does NOT make it true.

Here is somewhat of a checklist on where and how you can find reliable information when conducting internet searches. This will help you in becoming a well-informed, continual learner that is a capable self-advocate. If the website does not

These steps represent a complete package that must be used in combination. Make sure to use all of them as you review information that you receive from someone else or find online.

meet the first requirement, follow the checklist until it meets quality expectations. If it doesn't, it should be passed over for a more reputable source of information.

1. **What is the source of the website?**

   Hospital and government websites are trustworthy resources that provide accurate and current information to the readers. Examples of hospital websites include the Mayo Clinic and Cleveland Clinic. Examples of government websites include the NIH (National Institutes of Health), FDA (Food & Drug Administration), and CDC (Centers for Disease Control). Other websites can also be trustworthy, but must be further reviewed for confirmation.

2. **What are the credentials of the authors?**

   What training allows them to speak as authorities on the topic? You are likely familiar with many doctoral credentials, such as an MD, PharmD, or PhD. If you are unfamiliar with the credentials that you find, look them up! If admission for that program is easy and schooling is short, you might want to think twice about how much someone can really learn from such a program in that time. If the credential is not recognized by any licensing authorities, that is also a reason to pause. For instance, a doctor cannot practice just with an MD - he or she must also pass examinations and complete practical training in order to obtain a license to practice.

   If the authors do not have any credentials, then be wary of information that may be nothing more than speculation based off of one person's experience, or the result of a misunderstood comment or rumor. These are often found on support groups and blogs and can be equivalent to a dangerous game of Telephone or Whisper-Down-the-Lane.

3. **Do the authors speak within their credentials?**

I'm a pharmacist, and while that gives me significant room to speak about medications, therapies, and tests, it does not allow me to diagnose somebody or develop a diet and exercise plan for them. Similarly, a registered dietician is highly qualified to recommend diet and exercise, but cannot speak to medications and tests.

Be aware of the specialty of the credential. For instance, PhDs can be obtained in a variety of subjects, and just having a PhD does not mean that person is an expert on the topic that they are discussing. A PhD in Biochemistry does not educate a person on the topic of Psychology. I mentioned above that credentials should be recognized by licensing authorities. These licensing authorities authorize individuals to provide medical advice if they hold board certification, registration, or licensure. These individuals must abide by set standards to practice within their scope and avoid criminal charges.

4. **What does the author have to gain from writing about this?**

Conflicts of interest are an unfortunately common occurrence in this day and age. A conflict of interest occurs when a person that is providing advice or information has something to gain by providing it, whether that be prestige, money, perks, or otherwise. Information that is provided in the course of someone's paid position is less likely to be impacted by these conflicts, such as a dietician that is an employee of your health care system.

Websites that provide information free of charge are also likely to be unbiased and with good intention. However, beware of posts or websites that seem to promote specific products, or that discuss a topic and recommend only one specific treatment or product. It is not uncommon for bloggers to receive payment or free products in return for writing such articles and posts. While the writer may not intend any harm, this type of influence can alter what they write to overlook the negative and only emphasize the positive.

An author who is making an effort to remain unbiased and honest with his audience on a topic will always disclose any potential conflicts of interest.

5. What resources did that website use to find that information?

Is the resource only personal experience? It never hurts to learn about someone's personal experience – in fact, this is often incredibly helpful. However, it is impossible for one person's situation to be exactly the same as someone else's, particularly with a condition that is as variable as gastroparesis. The person writing the article or post should know this, and should make a statement to this effect. Always be cautious about applying someone else's experience to your own situation.

Do they make claims that they don't reference? If any statements are made as fact, or any comments are made such as "studies show...", then there should be a reference attached to this. If there is not, think twice before trusting that information. When references are available, always check that the references are reputable sources, such as medical journal articles, textbooks, or governmental websites.

As I said before, the internet is a powerful resource. That power is only magnified when given the tools to use it wisely and seek out only the most beneficial and valid information. If you are always a responsible consumer of information, then it will allow you to be responsible for and an active participant in your health.

EVIDENCE AND ANECDOTE

Another important point I would like to discuss regarding information is the difference between evidence and anecdote. It is very easy for someone who is well-intentioned to become wrapped up in a story or experience. When this happens, that person may begin to think that it applies to everyone, or at least to most people. This is the danger of the anecdote. In medical circles, it is sometimes called the "N of 1".

When I use the term "evidence", I am referring to large quantities of analyzed information that show a strong correlation, as well as a cause and effect. When this is missing, it is easy to confuse an unclear association with a true case of cause and effect. The classic example of a misinterpreted association is a study showing that when people consume ice cream at a higher rate, home break-ins increase. In this case, the wrong association is clearly wrong – it's hard to believe that something about the consumption of ice cream leads to aberrant behavior. In fact, it is simply that the rates of home break-ins are higher when the weather is warmer, which also happens to be the time when people are inclined to eat ice cream in larger quantities. Many, less obvious cases of mistaking an association for cause and effect exist in medicine and health. We will talk about some of these as we continue.

The term "N of 1" is shorthand for saying that the group that was used to develop a conclusion only included ONE person (n = 1).

All humans have a tendency to cling to the hope that lives in that one time or that one situation. Doctors are also inclined to remember that one patient that had a great outcome, even though they saw many others that did not.

Association: Two items, events, or topics appear to be connected in some way, although the nature of that connection is unclear.

Cause and Effect: One of two items in an association is clearly the reason for the occurrence or existence of the other item.

LEVELS OF EVIDENCE

There are a variety of sources for information and guidance that can be considered evidence in medicine. No matter how reputable the individual, if the evidence is lacking, then the recommendation may not be very safe, helpful, or reliable. Thus, it is important to understand the basics of sources of information in order to recognize how much support there is for the advice that is being given.

Medical guidance is often broken down into "Levels of Evidence". For demonstration purposes, these levels would look something like this:

1. Highly Supported
2. Supported
3. Promising
4. Unclear
5. Unsupported
6. Harmful

These levels of evidence depend on the number of studies that have been conducted on that topic and something called the robustness of the study. A study that was not conducted well or structured well would not increase the level of evidence. A study that had poor outcomes or showed that a certain recommendation may be harmful would skew the level of evidence towards #6.

Studies come in all shapes and sizes. Since I am a pharmacist and I can't help myself, my examples will generally include drugs. But the concepts apply to studies of all kinds, including medical devices (such as a pacemaker), surgeries, lifestyle changes, diet modifications, and more.

Randomized: Randomly places participants into different arms of the study

Controlled: Includes a 'control' arm that does not use the intervention that is being studied. This allows us to evaluate if it is the Intervention making a difference or some other cause.

Studies for medications for common illnesses such as heart disease will include thousands of people and will be in a format known as a Randomized Controlled Trial (RCT). RCTs are considered the gold standard because they are capable of demonstrating cause and effect. In these studies, there will be a group that is considered the "control group" that will either continue life as usual or take a placebo, and a group that is called the "treatment group" that will receive the studied treatment. These studies are good for answering a question like "If someone takes X drug, will they have less risk of Y?" or "If someone takes X drug, will they have less of Y symptom?".

The details of the study matter as well. The people that were enrolled in the study should represent the general population (male and female, multiracial, various ages, etc). The length of the study should allow enough time to see an impact (or lack thereof), to see if the impact continues over time or wears off, and to see if there are any unwanted side effects. Although they are never the primary goal of these RCTs, side effects and harmful outcomes are always monitored.

An RCT with thousands of people would provide what is considered #1, or Highly Supported evidence. Having more than one RCT that had the same results is even better. The larger the studies and the more people that were involved, the stronger the evidence that allows us to say "X should be used for Y". This goes all the way back to learning about the scientific method in school. Larger numbers and more repeats mean that the outcome is reproducible. In other words, it shows that X leads to Y the majority of the time, in the majority of situations. Or, conversely, that X does not lead to Y.

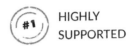 HIGHLY SUPPORTED

Unfortunately, most studies are not that large, and many of them are also not RCTs. From there, researchers and doctors move through studies that provide lower and lower categories of evidence. Some studies might be something called cohort studies. These review different populations of people and attempt to identify if the one difference between those populations resulted in Y (i.e. one population used this drug and the other didn't. Did the first population have more of Z?). These studies are often very large, but cannot always define a cause and effect relationship. Thus, they are considered the next best thing to RCTs.

Cohort: A group of people that share a certain characteristic and are followed through time.

These can include people that made a specific change (dietary, medication, etc.), that all have the same condition, that all completed a survey a certain way, and more. They are compared to a group of people that don't have this distinguishing feature.

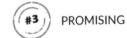 SUPPORTED

Other studies might go back and review existing information. These are called retrospective studies and are useful when they involve a lot of people and no other studies are available. However, they are prone to error because they rely on information that was already collected, so certain data may be missing or unclear. An example of this type of study is when someone reviews medical charts from a hospital visit that happened two years ago.

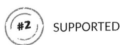 PROMISING

PROMISING #3

Other studies might collect information in different ways, including surveys and interviews. This information isn't considered quite as reliable for recommendations because it is subjective. However, it can be very useful for other purposes, such as clarifying the most common symptoms of a certain disease or the experiences of those that have a specific diagnosis. Again, the number of people involved is crucial. When numbers get smaller, it becomes much more difficult to draw accurate conclusions.

ANECDOTE

UNCLEAR #4

UNSUPPORTED #5

Case series and case reports are terms that are considered 'anecdotal evidence'. This means that the authors are reporting on the results of individual situations. While these studies may have importance for very rare diseases, they are an unreliable source of evidence, and would fall into categories #4 or #5. Medical recommendations should almost never come from this level of evidence.

Another form of anecdotal evidence is personal experience. This is found pretty commonly online and when not presented appropriately, can be misleading and even dangerous. When something happens to one person one time, it could be the result of chance or coincidence. That is why science is based on studies that show the outcome happens over and over again in different situations. When someone uses their personal experience as the foundation for advice and recommendations, they could be basing it on nothing more than a lucky coincidence. They could also be ignoring the fact that what worked for them may be very harmful to someone else.

In this book, I will be sharing my personal experiences in order to give an example of my own journey with gastroparesis and some ideas on coping strategies. However, I will never make a treatment recommendation or provide advice based solely on my experience. Be very wary of any resources that provide recommendations based on personal experience alone. Even the experience of a small group of people combined is still considered anecdotal and should be used with great caution.

EVIDENCE AND TIME

It is true that much of what we consider "Western medicine" is constantly changing and evolving. No doctor will tell you that we have perfected the treatment or testing for any disease at this point in time. Medicine is a learning field, meaning that each new experience adds valuable information to the knowledge bank, and that may eventually lead to a change in practice. In fact, modern medicine as we know it has existed for less than 100 years. It was only during this time that the field made a commitment to first observing and understanding disease and then scientifically evaluating possible therapies.

That's really a crazy thought! We didn't have a way to treat cancer, heart disease, or even an infected cut just 100 years ago. When put in that context, medicine has grown by leaps and bounds!

There are a number of reasons that medicine and the evidence behind it are constantly changing. One of these reasons is purely numbers-based. As more people develop heart disease, the profession gains more experience with treating and preventing it, and our treatments and prevention methods become better over time. This goes right back to the topic of Levels of Evidence. Larger numbers indicate reproducibility and better recommendations.

Another great example of the changing face of medicine is the use of antibiotics for the treatment of infections. Some antibiotics that used to be very effective are now only useful for a limited number of infections, such as penicillin. This is because our use of antibiotics over the past few decades has allowed bacteria to become resistant. Now, we are having to change our mindset about how and when to use which antibiotics, and the pharmaceutical industry is frantically searching for new drugs to which bacteria cannot become resistant. So while we might have thought we had that all figured out a couple of decades ago, that is no longer the case.

A less forgivable reason involves the misuse of evidence. Poor recommendations are often made as a result of a desire to provide answers when none are available. For instance, recent controversy has erupted over studies that show that the United States Nutrition Guidelines are wrong. We are just now finding out that calcium intake does not prevent fractures, and also finding out that our salt intake is lower than it should be. This is because the guidelines that we have used for decades were actually based off of poor levels of evidence. If the guidelines had held a higher standard for evidence and had simply made no recommendations at the time, then we could have waited for the large, high-quality studies that have recently been completed.

In a similar sense, fad diets and catchy lifestyle changes are often not all that they claim to be. They will eventually be replaced with the "next thing" and may even be shown to be harmful or useless. When new studies pop up in the media, it is often best to wait for them to be reviewed by the medical community, or even for other studies to confirm the findings.

A particularly relevant example of a small study being blown out of proportion is the study that launched the national concern over gluten sensitivity. For all of the media attention that this study gained, it only involved 34 people. The physician that conducted the study is a good scientist, and he went back to confirm his own results. What he found in his later, more robustly structured study, was that gluten sensitivity was not truly present. However, at that point, the media had elevated gluten to the level of a public enemy and the results of his later studies were ignored. We now know much more about who will and will not benefit from a gluten-free diet. But as a response to the media running with the first story, millions of people have dramatically altered their diets and possibly become less healthy because of it.

Don't worry, there is much more to come on this topic later, and we will review the newer information that has become available.

It is also important to understand that guidelines, such as nutritional guidelines, are based off of a summary of the evidence that is out there. Some guidelines are better than others and some utilize higher standards of evidence than others. This is helpful to remember when trying to incorporate this information into your own life. If a specific number is stated as a goal, a range is acceptable instead. For instance, a goal of 25 grams of fat could be interpreted more loosely as 20–30 grams.

Trying to stick to a single number instead of a range is kind of like believing that the passing of a single day suddenly provides the mental capacity to drive, vote, drink alcohol, or rent a car.

SELECTING CHANGES TO TRY

I realize that this was a lot of uncertainty to throw together all at once and leaves the very important question of "How do I apply this?" There are admittedly a number of factors to consider with any recommendation or advice. But all of these factors can be applied in just a few steps.

1. **Be discriminatory about where you obtain your advice and recommendations.**

   If it came from a source that may not be very knowledgeable or may have accidentally misunderstood something that they heard, verify it! The steps to do so can be found at the beginning of this chapter. If you filter out the information that is not helpful and the advice that is not likely to get you anywhere, it allows you to focus your energy where it matters.

2. **Use common sense when reading about a new treatment or idea**

   If it claims to fix a wide variety of issues, it is almost definitely too good to be true. If it is a concept that would be worth billions of dollars to a drug company and yet no one is developing or marketing it, then it is probably too good to be true. This might be because it doesn't work or because it is too dangerous to justify using. The information that we will cover throughout this book will give you the knowledge to recognize more situations and concepts that don't make sense or sound too good to be true.

3. Consider if it truly makes sense for you, your symptoms, and your lifestyle

It's easy to jump at any hope for improvement, but sometimes those hopes don't even address the symptoms that are impacting you the most. Or sometimes they are just too difficult to implement to make them worthwhile due to the change in lifestyle or the way they make you feel.

It can be easy to become overwhelmed with ideas and possible changes to make, which can sometimes strand people in a state of inaction. Filtering down to only those options that have the most evidence and promise for you will allow for better focus, but there might still be quite a few!

IMPLEMENTING SELECTED CHANGES

This is where we all fall into the trap of trying to do everything at once. The problem with this is that if something is hurting us OR making us better, we will never know which change is doing what. That is a very frustrating feeling. And it's scary to know that something is working and then have to slowly start peeling away changes to find the cause, wondering if the things that you are taking away might lead to a relapse. Throwing the kitchen sink at a problem like gastroparesis is always incredibly tempting (and I've done it), but not very useful in the long run.

A careful and planned approach will be immensely helpful in the long term. It will let you know definitively what does and does not work for you. It will allow you to tweak things to fit you specifically and move on from ideas that just aren't cutting it.

The initial step would be to order the changes such that the first ones represent the options that you believe are most likely to help and that you are most excited about – you should try those first. However, only one change should be tried at a time.

Find out how long it is supposed to take to recognize a difference and plan to try it for at least that long. For instance, some medications can take up to 6–8 weeks to have their full effect, whereas a change in preparation of a specific food item could result in almost immediate effect. Also, be aware of what can go wrong with each change, and be vigilant in your awareness of those possibilities. This could include a new diet that might make you more gassy, or a medication that causes you to feel exhausted all of the time. As we move through this book, we will cover many of the tools and resources that can be used to identify and apply this information.

What must be considered when making a change:

1. Possible side effects
2. Possible benefits
3. How long it will take to see a difference
4. How long to test the change before being able to decide if it is helping or hurting

Knowing what to expect going in and trying each change separately will allow you to identify the presence of issues that make you feel worse (such as exhaustion caused by a medication or a poor diet). Recognizing these issues can allow you to decide to move on to another option instead. You will also be able to say with assurance that a change made a positive difference and that you would like to continue it as you add on another change.

SUMMARY

Everything that we have covered in this chapter will be integrated into the many topics discussed throughout the rest of the book. Stamps will appear in the margins to indicate the level of evidence for the information being discussed. The considerations that should be made for evaluating your sources and new ideas will also be broken down further and applied to specific situations.

Although paring through levels of evidence and evaluating resources may seem like a daunting task, it will begin to feel comfortable and straightforward as we apply these concepts to topics that directly affect each of us with gastroparesis. We now have one tool that we will integrate with many others as we develop our roadmaps.

The Gastrointestinal System

3

Something that I have never been able to find in all of my searches is a description of the GI tract that speaks to someone with gastroparesis. Every description always seems to be missing an important component, whether it's too basic, too complex, or just not focused enough on issues with motility. And even though doctors often only talk about your upper GI tract, all portions end up playing a role in gastroparesis symptoms.

In order to really understand this condition and the ways to manage it, we must understand what is happening. So, I would like to spend just a little bit of time reviewing the nuts and bolts of the GI tract. I will refer back to this many times during discussions on symptoms and treatment.

GI TRACT FUNCTION

DIGESTION

The GI tract is primarily known for its role in digestion. For our purposes, there are two main types of digestion that occur in the GI tract. These are mechanical and chemical. Mechanical implies physical impact on the food/substances that are passing through the GI tract. This can be in the form of chewing and also in the form of the stomach grinding down its contents. Chemical implies that some type of substance in the body is breaking down the food at the molecular level. This happens in multiple parts of the GI tract with various types of fluids, such as stomach acid.

ABSORPTION

The whole purpose of taking in food (besides the fact that it tastes good!) is to provide our bodies with nutrition, so a primary role of the GI tract is to absorb the nutrients that are found in the foods that we eat. Absorption occurs in various parts of the GI tract, but can only be completed once digestion has taken place and broken the food down into smaller components. Our bodies have developed a variety of interesting and creative ways of accessing the nutrients that we consume.

EXCRETION

The GI tract is also quite well known for its role in ridding our bodies of waste in the form of stool. Many actions occur that lead to the proper formation of stool that is not too hard and not too soft. This all happens after, hopefully, the nutrients and water in the food that was consumed have been properly absorbed by the body.

OTHER FUNCTIONS

As the GI tract has become the subject of renewed research and interest, a number of additional functions have recently been attributed to this complex part of our bodies. It has now become clear that the GI tract is actually the largest component of the body's immune system. It also seems to be the case that the human GI tract plays a large role in the endocrine system. These findings are just the beginning of an evolving field of science that will probably lead to a large shift in the way that we view our GI tracts. However, for the sake of gastroparesis, we are mostly concerned with the digestion, absorption, and excretion functions of our guts.

Endocrine System:
A collection of glands that transmits signals and secretes hormones into the blood stream to be carried to other parts of the body.

THE GASTROINTESTINAL SYSTEM

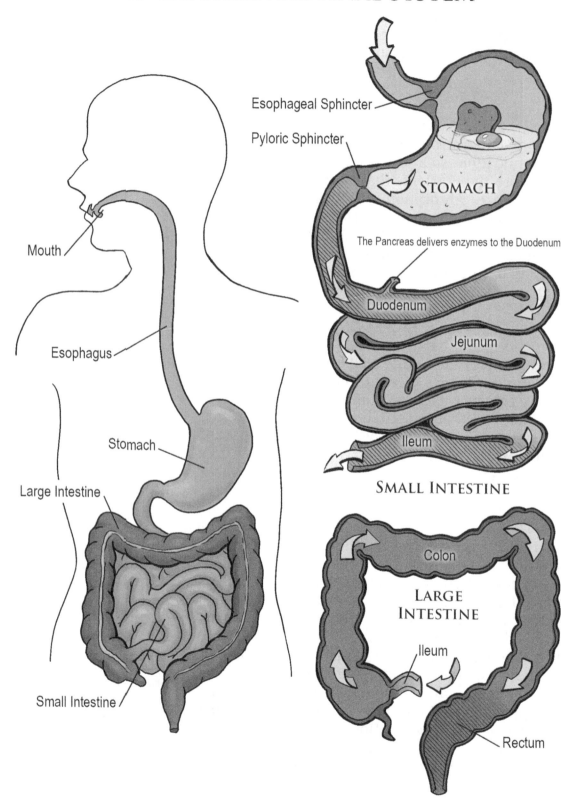

Esophageal Sphincter

Pyloric Sphincter

STOMACH

The Pancreas delivers enzymes to the Duodenum

Duodenum

Jejunum

Ileum

SMALL INTESTINE

Mouth

Esophagus

Stomach

Large Intestine

Small Intestine

Colon

LARGE INTESTINE

Ileum

Rectum

GI TRACT STRUCTURE

MOUTH

The mouth is where digestion begins, starting with chemical breakdown from saliva and mechanical breakdown from chewing. There are also some medications that are partially absorbed in the mouth. This is why there is sometimes the option to have an orally disintegrating tablet instead of a tablet that is swallowed. It isn't possible for all medications, but the medications that are made this way have been shown to have good absorption in the mouth.

ESOPHAGUS

Once the food passes through the mouth, it is swallowed and travels down the esophagus. This is where something called peristalsis comes in. Peristalsis is made up of involuntary contractions. In other words, muscles in your body are supposed to be constantly moving in a direction that pushes the food down the esophagus and into the stomach. Once in the stomach, peristalsis causes the stomach to move around and perform mechanical digestion. There are a number of things that can go wrong here, including unregulated movement, which might cause the food to get stuck or move the wrong direction, or the complete lack of peristalsis, which means that there is no movement at all.

ESOPHAGEAL SPHINCTER

The gateway between the esophagus and the stomach is called the esophageal sphincter. This is a flap that keeps the food moving in only one direction: esophagus to stomach. When there is a vomiting reflex, it overrides this sphincter and pushes food back into the esophagus. There are also other issues that can occur with this sphincter. Due to certain foods or medications, it can become loose, which allows food to leak past it in the wrong direction. For others, the sphincter can actually become completely ineffective, which leaves an opening for food to move in both directions relatively freely. Many people with gastroparesis experience regurgitation without a vomiting reflex, which indicates they likely have some type of esophageal sphincter malfunction.

STOMACH

Mechanical and chemical digestion occur inside of the stomach. This happens through movement of the stomach as well as through the presence of stomach acid. There is a distinct difference between the acid that is produced by the stomach on a regular basis and the acids that come from the food that has been eaten. Stomach acid is a popular topic for people with gastroparesis, and we will discuss this in more detail later on. The stomach is considered the hub for the symptoms of gastroparesis. For whatever reason (and these can vary), there is an increase in the time it takes for the food to empty out of the stomach. This is popularly referred to as gastric emptying time and everyone with a gastroparesis diagnosis has likely had this test at least once. The time it takes for the stomach to empty its contents is key to a gastroparesis diagnosis.

The term "emptying time" will be discussed and explained in the next chapter.

PYLORIC SPHINCTER

Once the food is adequately broken down to a liquid form, it drains out of the stomach through the pyloric sphincter. Just as with the last sphincter, this one also works to keep the contents of the GI tract moving in only one direction: stomach to small intestine. This sphincter does not suffer from the malfunctions that are seen with the esophageal sphincter nearly as often, and that usually does not play into the symptoms for someone with gastroparesis. However, a different issue with this sphincter has been found to exacerbate gastroparesis for some people – tightening. If the pyloric sphincter is too tight, it is difficult for food to drain out of the stomach at an adequate rate, leading to delayed gastric emptying.

DUODENUM

The small intestine is made up of three pieces, called the duodenum, jejunum, and ileum, in that order. The first two terms might sound familiar for some people because they are commonly used when discussing feeding tubes. These are the tubes that are sometimes placed in order to provide food to the body without using the stomach. We will go into more detail on different feeding options in a later chapter.

From the pyloric sphincter, the food enters the duodenum. The nutrients in the food that has been eaten are now broken down by enzymes so that they can be absorbed and used by the body. This breakdown and absorption continues throughout the small intestine, and we will look at each of its pieces separately.

PANCREAS

Enzymes for nutrient breakdown come from the pancreas and are referred to, understandably, as pancreatic enzymes. The primary components here are enzymes that break down fats, proteins, and carbohydrates (sugars). Additional enzymes break down fibers and other nutrients that may be difficult to digest. These enzymes are delivered to the duodenum and mixed with the digested food that has exited the stomach. Something called sodium bicarbonate is also released from the pancreas into the duodenum. This chemical deactivates the acid that was mixed with the food while in the stomach.

This is a departure from the other components that we have discussed because our food does not actually pass through the pancreas. However, I've included it here because this organ is crucial to the function of the GI tract and feeds directly into the small intestine. The pancreas is more well-known for its role in diabetes and producing insulin.

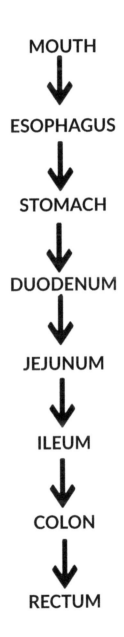

MOUTH
↓
ESOPHAGUS
↓
STOMACH
↓
DUODENUM
↓
JEJUNUM
↓
ILEUM
↓
COLON
↓
RECTUM

JEJUNUM

From the duodenum, the food moves into the next section of the small intestine – the jejunum. The jejunum's primary function is the absorption of the nutrients in the food. It is full of cells that pull the nutrients into the body. The goal is to leave nothing valuable in the intestine – it should only end up with indigestible and nutrient-free waste. The jejunum is also important in absorbing water into the body. Once nutrients are absorbed they are typically processed by the liver, but we will not discuss this processing in any detail here.

ILEUM

After the jejunum, the food passes into the next part of the intestine called the ileum. The ileum basically acts as the cleanup for nutrient absorption. It picks up anything that was not absorbed by the jejunum, and is responsible for absorbing specific nutrients that the jejunum cannot absorb. The ileum is also responsible for absorbing water into the body.

Keep in mind that peristalsis is active in the intestine as well as in the esophagus and stomach. Muscle contractions are responsible for keeping food and stool moving towards the rectum all the way through the intestine. And for some people, while peristalsis may be disrupted in the upper GI tract (esophagus and stomach), it is quite normal in the intestine. This is important for combatting another hot topic for those of us with gastroparesis – constipation.

COLON

After completing its run through the small intestine, food, which is now called chyme, is moved into the large intestine through a passage called the cecum. The large intestine is also called the colon and is broken into a few different segments. The colon is responsible for removing the last bits of nutrients and also any extra water from the chyme. Certain vitamins are produced by the bacteria found in the colon, and are absorbed from this location (such as Vitamin K, Vitamin B12, Vitamin B1 or thiamine, and Vitamin B2 or riboflavin).

RECTUM

Finally, the food makes its way to the rectum, where it is stored until it exits the body through the anus. And as we are all aware, stool can come in many forms, from fully liquid to very hard and solid, and the causes of these changes in its forms are numerous. We will cover as many of these as possible later in this book.

BACTERIA AND OUR BODIES

There has been a lot of press in recent years regarding the human microbiome or gut bacteria. It is true that our bodies are home to trillions of tiny organisms, and the majority of these live in our GI tract. There are some in our mouths, in our stomachs, and throughout the different parts of the small and large intestine. While many of these bacteria serve a beneficial purpose and function for our bodies, some of them do not.

A trillion = 1,000,000,000,000

The research on the microbiome is ongoing, and there is still a lot that we don't know. Some of the things that we thought we knew years ago have now been shown to be wrong, so it's important to not jump too quickly at any news that breaks regarding this topic. When there are trillions of organisms hanging out, there is a lot of information to be aware of in order to fully understand how something might impact you. But it does seem clear that the GI tract and its bacteria have impacts that we never would have expected, including to our immune systems and on the development of allergies.

Microbiome:
The collection of microorganisms found within a particular environment (in this case, the gut)

Many different types of bacteria are located all over our bodies. Some of you might have had a dental procedure in the past and the dentist may have prescribed an antibiotic. This isn't because he was worried about infecting you during the surgery. It's actually because he was worried that the bacteria living in your mouth might get into your blood where it doesn't belong. In fact, many people don't realize that it is the bacteria that is always present on our skin that causes most of the infections in the little scrapes and cuts that we get in our everyday lives. When our bacteria stay where they are supposed to, they benefit us. But sometimes they go where they are not supposed to, and that other part of our body is not equipped to deal with that type of bacteria.

BACTERIA IN THE GUT

When a baby is born, there is no bacteria found in his or her gut. However, within about 48 hours, the gut becomes filled with bacteria. These bacteria have been found to be different depending on whether the baby is breastfed or formula-fed. It is likely that this ties into some of the other conditions that are now being associated with breastfeeding versus formula-feeding, but that is a topic for another book! The important thing to note here is how sensitive the gut flora actually is to diet and environment. As humans grow older, our guts become less sensitive to these little changes, but larger and persistent changes can still make an impact on our microbiome.

There are 10 times more bacterial cells found in the gut than the number of cells in the entire human body. All combined, the gut bacteria would weigh about the same as your liver (~3.5 lbs)..

Different factors can affect the numbers and types of bacteria that live in our guts. Some of these factors cannot be changed, such as our ages, genders, and genetic inheritances. But other factors that have a large impact can be changed, such as infections and diet. Alterations to these factors can lead to GI symptoms, including bloating, pain, nausea, vomiting, diarrhea, constipation, and more.

FUNCTION

Believe it or not, the bacteria in our gut actually serve a purpose. They are present in a symbiotic relationship with our bodies. In other words, when we feed the bacteria that live in our gut, the bacteria give something helpful back in return.

This may come in the form of digestion – bacteria can sometimes be helpful in digesting substances that are difficult for our bodies to break down. This allows our bodies to absorb nutrients that we might not have been able to access otherwise. Different bacterial species will be capable of breaking down different items, so having a variety of species around increases our nutritional status.

Some bacteria produce substances that our bodies need. Bifidobacterium produces substances that help to bulk up our immune systems. Other bacteria actually produce some of the vitamins that we need to live, including Vitamin K (crucial for blood clotting) and the B Vitamin family. And still other bacteria even produce small fatty acids that the human body can use as an energy source!

But as you might expect, there are ways that this symbiotic relationship can go a little bit wrong. For instance, bacteria may sometimes produce air when they break down certain substances, which our bodies read as gas. It is also possible for bacteria that typically live in one part of the intestine to move to another part where they don't play as nicely. And still another possibility is for a bacteria that is not typically found in the GI tract at all to take up residence and shake things up. Thus, it is helpful to have an understanding for where we expect to find which bacteria, if any at all.

Studies of people in different parts of the world are showing that the bacteria in our guts might help to explain why some people can digest foods that others can't. Or why some groups of people are able to live off of seemingly limited diets but stay well-nourished, regardless.

Bacteria can evolve to break down different items and also to produce different types of nutrients from those items. It is an interesting and developing field of science, indeed!

BACTERIA THROUGHOUT THE GI TRACT

MOUTH

Various types of bacteria live all over our gums and teeth. They show up pretty quickly after we're born and never go away. These bacteria are credited with causing such nuisances as cavities and oral infections. Research is still being done to better understand the difference between 'healthy' and 'infectious' bacteria in the mouth. This is not as relevant to gastroparesis as the rest of the GI tract, but is still an interesting topic to consider.

STOMACH

The stomach is an incredibly acidic environment. It was previously thought to be fatal to all bacteria until a species called Helicobacter pylori (H. pylori) was discovered that is actually able to survive this environment. It is not a natural inhabitant of the human stomach, but humans can become colonized by it.

H. Pylori is NOT more common for those with gastroparesis, but if it happens it can make symptoms worse.

Infection with H. pylori is not more common in those with gastroparesis, but it can happen. This infection causes various symptoms which can then increase the level of discomfort someone with gastroparesis might be experiencing. These include stomach pain, increased nausea, decreased appetite, bloating, and weight loss. Anyone with gastroparesis can see how much these symptoms can overlap with what they are already experiencing.

The tests to check for H. pylori are very simple – breath and stool. Considering how much this infection can worsen the symptoms of gastroparesis, it makes sense for anyone with gastroparesis to have the test completed. Unfortunately, some medications that are used to suppress stomach acid may interfere with the tests, and must be stopped a couple of weeks prior to the test. This makes many people nervous, and we will get into full detail on this topic later.

SMALL INTESTINE

As we move into the small intestine, it becomes normal to see some bacteria, although not many. Only a few species of bacteria will be found, including names that are familiar to many people – lactobacillus and enterococcus. These bacteria are considered standard and beneficial to GI function. For some people, there may actually be no bacteria growing in parts of the small intestine, and this is fine.

The distal ileum is considered a 'transition' from the small intestine to the large intestine and more bacteria may be found here. This is also where bacteria can begin to creep into a space where they don't belong, leading to what has recently become a highly publicized condition - Small Intestinal Bacterial Overgrowth (SIBO). SIBO occurs when bacteria that are normal and appropriate in the large intestine work their way into the small intestine where they don't belong and are not as well tolerated. A much larger discussion will be dedicated to this topic later in the book.

Small Intestinal Bacterial Overgrowth (SIBO):
Bacteria that are moving in the wrong direction – from the large intestine to the small intestine

LARGE INTESTINE

The large intestine is home to the variety of bacteria that are often discussed when references are made to the gut flora or the human microbiome. It is believed there may be as many as 500–1,000 species living in our guts, and a large portion of these have not been identified. The bacteria that help to digest our foods and produce important vitamins and components that improve our health are found in this part of the GI tract. Believe it or not, there are even some medications that are processed in part by the bacteria that live there.

DISRUPTION OF FUNCTION

A variety of factors can disrupt the regular function of the GI tract, particularly in relation to bacteria. Something as simple as taking antibiotics for an infection will actually kill off some of the bacteria in the gut. This change in the makeup of the gut flora causes some people to experience diarrhea when taking certain antibiotics.

I mentioned before that the stomach is typically free of bacteria because it is so acidic. This acidic environment has the added benefit of killing off any bacteria that might have been swallowed before they reach the intestine. Reducing the acidity of the stomach (which can happen by taking medications that suppress stomach acid) can increase the risk of having bacteria move into places where they should not be found.

Motility of the GI tract can also have an impact on keeping bacteria where they belong. The constant forward movement that results from peristalsis keeps bacteria moving down the GI tract and into the large intestine. When this is disrupted, it can also increase the chances of bacteria colonizing somewhere unusual. In a similar way, an intestinal obstruction or an unusually shaped intestine can have the same result.

The pancreas is responsible for excreting bile, which also has some antibiotic effects. This helps to keep the number of bacteria present in the small intestine to a minimum. Thus, having reduced pancreatic activity may also lead to bacteria taking up residence in an unusual location.

SUMMARY

We have now covered the basic structure and function of the GI tract and its many pieces, with a specific focus on motility and the processing and absorption of food. Understanding the inhabitants of the GI tract will also aid us in understanding the many concerns that can arise in relation to the bacteria that reside within us. This knowledge will now allow us to discuss GI-specific topics and issues on a deeper level.

What can go wrong with the bacteria in our guts:

1. Using certain medications, like antibiotics and acid reducers
2. Altering the natural environment in the gut
3. Disruptions in intestinal motility, both temporary and permanent
4. Functional changes in organs that are part of the GI system, but not the GI tract, such as the liver and pancreas

Personal Experience

At this point, I was in my first year of college and noticing my symptoms worsening with the week. I was bringing up every single thing that I ate, often over twelve hours later. If I ate something for dinner, I knew I would taste it again in the morning. I was learning that carbonated beverages did not shoot back up my throat the way that water did, and developed a soda addiction to replace what used to be a very healthy water habit.

My nausea was becoming increasingly present. I felt nauseated from the second I woke until the time that I went to bed. I developed a tolerance for it, but sometimes it would flare up enough to knock me flat and put me out of commission. I also had to be very careful to avoid sudden movements or any positions that could exacerbate the nausea. For all of my determination, I couldn't work or go to class when every tiny movement made me heave.

My stomach was constantly in pain - a pressure pain that never went away. I experienced incredible discomfort when anything pushed against my stomach, be it a tight waistline or an accidental bump. At times that constant pressure pain would evolve into a throbbing, concentrated pain that would distract me from whatever I was doing at the time. Doubling over at work and school is not a very fun experience, especially when it happens over and over again.

I became very constipated, gassy, and bloated at all times. My stomach felt like it had been inflated like a basketball. This was uncomfortable and also embarrassing to experience in college when I could not afford a new wardrobe to accommodate this change in shape.

Most concerning of all to me was the development of what I called the "shakes". This started out as a debilitating spell of shaking, and then progressed to also include fuzziness, dimness, and even fainting. There was no way for me to handle this without just waiting it out. My car became my refuge where I could lie down and feel horrible by myself, maybe even pass out without anyone needing to notice or help.

What all of this added up to was a very diminished quality of life at a time when I was supposed to be living it up. I was perpetually self-conscious and distracted by my entire GI tract, from top to bottom. I was also so very angry at the situation. I had always had a healthy diet and now I was eating horribly because nothing healthy seemed to go down. Why couldn't I just go out to eat like a normal person, or drink like a normal college student? How was it fair that I had to worry about throwing up without notice or passing out while standing at work? I was embarrassed by my appearance and worried that others would be able to see through me and know what I was experiencing and then treat me differently because of it.

While being angry at the injustice of it all, I was also despairing at the permanence and the prospects for my future.

Gastoparesis Basics 4

"The mind is like the stomach. It is not how much you put in that counts, but how much it digests."

ALBERT J. NOCK

Considering that this is a book about gastroparesis, we should probably start talking about that, right? Now that we have a strong understanding of the GI tract, it will be easier to discuss the nuts and bolts of gastroparesis. So here goes!

Motility is a very important feature to the proper function of the GI tract. When GI motility isn't working the way that it is supposed to, the GI tract can start to go a bit haywire as it attempts to conduct its three main functions: digestion, absorption, and excretion (see page 29).

We briefly discussed peristalsis in the previous section – the movement of the GI tract that pushes everything in the correct direction. This occurs through a series of muscle contractions that happen in a certain sequence from the esophagus to the large intestine. Beyond simply moving the food in the appropriate direction, peristalsis is responsible for the movement of the stomach as it churns up the food (mechanical digestion). It also helps our intestines to absorb nutrients more completely by moving the food along the wall of the intestine.

Peristalsis originates from a Greek term meaning "to wrap around"

DEFINING GASTROPARESIS

Gastroparesis is, very simply, a delay in the time that it takes for the contents of the stomach to

Gastroparesis is Greek for "partial paralysis of the stomach" empty into the intestine (see page 33). It usually indicates a disruption in gastric motility, or the peristalsis that we just discussed. For each person, the extent of the disruption in motility may be different, the extent of the delay may be different, and the symptoms that these issues cause are also typically different. But for the large majority of those with gastroparesis, the issues with motility are limited to portions of the upper GI tract, or specifically the esophagus and stomach.

Disruption of peristalsis could mean that there is no movement of the muscles, very limited movement of the muscles, or disordered movement of the muscles. These all come together to have the very similar effect of delaying the movement of food through the GI tract. Additionally, this disruption in peristalsis can occur in the esophagus, the stomach, or in both the esophagus and stomach. The extent and severity of the disruption can each contribute to a different presentation of the condition and a different array of symptoms.

It is currently very difficult to accurately state how many people have a gastroparesis diagnosis. Recent attempts have estimated an incidence rate of 6.3 per 100,000 persons per year, or around 5 million people in the United States. Another publication noted that the rate of hospitalization related to gastroparesis has increased in recent years, but it is unclear if this is because the rate of gastroparesis is increasing or simply because it is being diagnosed more accurately. On a similar note, there has been some discussion regarding the amount of undiagnosed gastroparesis that is likely present, but efforts to evaluate how large this population might actually be are primarily hypothetical in nature.

CAUSES OF GASTROPARESIS

Idiopathic is Greek for "one's own suffering"

There are many possible causes of gastroparesis. While in pursuit of trying to find the cause, most of us are told that it is idiopathic. This means that there is no clear reason that we developed this condition. It seems that a large number of those with idiopathic gastroparesis, myself included, had some type of viral illness right before it happened, but that is about the extent of our understanding. However, this form of gastroparesis is not any more difficult to treat or control than other forms.

The most common identified cause is diabetes. When someone with diabetes develops gastroparesis, it happens over a long period of time and is actually a complication of sugar imbalances in the body. The severity of the condition may be different for those with diabetic gastroparesis, but there are also many additional considerations, including the need to factor in diabetic dietary constraints.

Damage to the vagus nerve is another cause of gastroparesis. The vagus nerve is responsible for stimulating the muscle contractions in the stomach that allow for mechanical digestion. When this nerve is damaged, it can impair or eliminate these contractions. Incidentally, the sugar imbalances that lead to diabetic gastroparesis do so through damage to the vagus nerve. An illness can also damage the nerve, as well as a direct injury through some type of abdominal surgery.

Another, albeit uncommon, possibility is for gastroparesis to be the result of another chronic condition (other than diabetes) that has already been diagnosed. Some people with disorders that affect multiple parts of the body are simply more prone to the development of gastroparesis. This may be through a generalized nerve or muscle malfunction, or through another mechanism entirely. Ehrlos-Danlos Syndrome and Mitochondrial Disorders are two rare disorders that can sometimes produce gastroparesis.

SYMPTOMS OF GASTROPARESIS

Gastroparesis is a strange condition in that every person not only has a slightly different set of

When you read about gastroparesis symptoms online, it can sometimes be confusing because they won't necessarily align with yours. Gastroparesis presents very differently for different people, and your doctor should listen to your specific concerns, even if he wasn't expecting all of them.

I never knew how much I took hunger for granted until it was gone.

I personally have chronic regurgitation. Once I start eating, I know my food is going to travel back up and down as it pleases throughout the day. This was at first a horrible experience and very difficult to manage (i.e. while holding a conversation), but over time I have forgotten what it is like to NOT have my food regurgitate. Strange how we adapt...

symptoms, but each person may also experience the symptoms at different times. We discussed that the extent and location of the motility issues were partly responsible for this variation, but there are a number of other factors that can have an impact on symptom presentation, and we will touch on many of these throughout the book.

As you might expect when food doesn't move properly through the GI tract, one of the primary symptoms of gastroparesis is a feeling of fullness. This symptom causes another common 'complication' for those with gastroparesis – a loss of their sense of hunger. Food can hang around for quite some time, which can tack on some additional symptoms. These might include acid reflux, regurgitation, nausea, vomiting, bloating, pain, and more. As the reduced motility in the upper GI tract causes changes in the way that the food is processed, other issues can arise lower down in the GI tract, including sugar imbalances, cramping, diarrhea, constipation, and gas.

I want to quickly explain the difference between two things that sound similar but are actually quite different – regurgitation and vomiting. Many doctors throw these words out as though everyone knows their meaning, but I remember being at a loss when I first heard these terms used together.

Regurgitation is the involuntary reflux of food back up through the esophagus and sometimes into the mouth. It does not rely on any type of nausea stimulus and does not even involve a heaving motion. The food just finds its way back up whether you like it or not! Another important thing to point out is that the food that comes up may actually be undigested and very similar to the form it was in when it went down. It is only after it has been in the stomach for an extended period of time that it becomes acidic and harsh on the throat and mouth.

Vomiting is the type of reflux that we are more used to experiencing and hearing about outside of gastroparesis. This usually involves a lot of nausea and always involves a painful and exhausting heaving motion in which the muscles actively push food back up through the esophagus and into the mouth. While the food that is brought up through vomiting may also be primarily undigested and non-acidic due to only being in the stomach for a short period of time, vomiting is more likely than regurgitation to produce a substance that is digested and acidic, which is harsh on the throat and mouth.

A person with gastroparesis can experience regurgitation, vomiting, or both. In addition, people with regurgitation can experience nausea that does not often lead to vomiting. But if a doctor is trying to get a clear picture of your symptoms, you can now provide an accurate answer regarding how severely and how often each of those things happens for you (if at all).

The symptoms that people experience can also be very different as far as when they appear. Some people with gastroparesis will experience chronic symptoms that are always present and may worsen at certain times. Others will only experience symptoms periodically. Some people refer to these as symptom 'flares' and they can typically be associated with stress, diet, or illness. The fluctuation in symptom presence and severity can lead to an unexpected complication for some people – anxiety. We will have a more in-depth discussion regarding anxiety and stress and how it plays into gastroparesis symptoms later in the book.

DIAGNOSIS AND TESTING OF GASTROPARESIS

THE EMPTYING TEST

Most people that have a gastroparesis diagnosis have gone through everyone's favorite test – the gastric emptying test (or officially, gastric emptying scintigraphy). This is really considered the

EMPTYING TEST VISUALIZED

START

100% of food in stomach

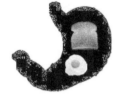

AFTER 4 HOURS...

NORMAL

<10% of food left at Hour 4 (>90% gone)

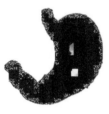

DELAYED

>10% of food left at Hour 4 (<90% gone)

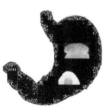

gold standard for diagnosing gastroparesis. As you are likely familiar, the test involves the consumption of eggs and a piece of toast with jelly on it. The eggs have a radioactive substance added to them that can be scanned as it passes through the GI tract. There are different lengths of time for this test ranging from 2 to 6 hours. Each doctor will have their own preference, but the test that is considered to be the standard is the 4-hour test.

This test is very simplistic in that it tells you how much food has emptied out of your stomach and into your small intestine in a certain length of time. This is reported in a percentage, with the normal range usually considered to be 90% of food exiting the stomach in 4 hours. Anything less than that is considered delayed, with the lower percentages indicating a more severe delay. It is interesting to point out that the severity of the delay does not always seem to be associated with the severity of symptoms. Some people with extensive delay may not feel as sick as those with more minor delays.

UPPER ENDOSCOPY

This is not really considered a diagnostic test so much as a way for the doctor to get a better understanding for the state of your upper GI tract. With this test, the doctor will place a camera down your throat and be able to examine your esophagus and stomach. While he is doing this, he is able to visually assess motility in both of these areas. He can evaluate the condition of your sphincters (esophageal and pyloric) for looseness and tightness (see page 32). He is also able to look for any other concerns, such as ulcers, hernias, or blockages. Finally, he can even collect a sample that allows him to test your stomach for H. pylori (see page 38).

This procedure requires the use of a small amount of sedation that allows placement of the tube down your throat. Luckily that sedation also causes amnesia, so you don't have to remember the experience once it is over. But that also means you might repeat yourself a few times as you come out of the haze!

BARIUM TESTING

Barium is a very interesting product because even though it is used for imaging, it is not actually radioactive. Instead, it is a substance that x-rays cannot pass through, which makes it stand out loud and clear on scans. In this case, it coats the walls of the GI tract, allowing the doctor to visualize the flow and shape of your GI tract.

This test can be done in a few ways. The quickest version, the swallow test, involves simply tracing the barium down the esophagus to assess for any structural issues. A lengthier version is called the Upper GI Series, which involves the coating of the entire stomach. This does require some rolling and flipping, and possibly some uncomfortable placement of a pad under the stomach as needed for imaging. Finally, a doctor might be interested in seeing the passage of the barium through the small intestine. This is the longest version of the test and once the scanning of the stomach is complete, it is simply a waiting game.

This test requires you to swallow a lot of barium, which is a kind of chalky, milky substance. You may be asked to swallow effervescent barium as well, which produces a barium gas in the stomach to visualize the entire organ. As you might imagine, the production of the gas in the stomach does cause significant burping. Both of these products may cause nausea for people with gastroparesis, but it is limited. Finally, when you pass the barium in your stool, it will appear pale and white, which can be concerning if you are not prepared for it.

When I had my Upper GI Series, I was laying in front of three medical residents and the attending physician and wearing a thin, poorly tied hospital gown. I was mortified and spent the entire time trying to hold the gown together while rolling as requested.

I wish I had known then that I could have spoken up. I could have asked to have the medical residents leave the room. I could have asked for another gown to provide better coverage.

Never be afraid to speak up for yourself and never assume that you should just "deal with it".

ESOPHAGEAL MANOMETRY

This test involves the placement of a tube down the nose and into the esophagus and stomach. The tube is then able to evaluate the muscle contractions inside of the esophagus at various points.

The test can be more or less extensive depending on what the doctor hopes to evaluate while the tube is placed. The pressure and muscle activity can be evaluated at rest, evaluated with the consumption of food or liquids, and also evaluated in response to different medications.

The actual placement of the tube through the nose can be uncomfortable and difficult, but once it is in place, it is typically only a mild discomfort. Each person's experience with esophageal manometry is different depending on the extent of what the doctor is planning to observe and how well you are feeling on the day it is conducted. This is a less common test to have performed and not everyone with gastroparesis will have one completed.

OTHER TESTS

Some other tests may be conducted depending on how you contracted gastroparesis or because the doctor wants to rule out other possible causes first. For instance, further imaging of the abdomen may be done in order to make sure that there are no issues with the pancreas or gallbladder. Blood tests may be conducted to look for underlying causes like diabetes or an underactive thyroid. Some people may even swallow something called a SmartPill that keeps data on how quickly it moves through different parts of the GI tract.

Gastroparesis in babies and small children is very different than what is experienced by adults and often resolves slowly with normal growth through childhood. The challenge is for them to get adequate nutrition to allow for this normal growth.

When very small children are being assessed for gastroparesis, they sometimes undergo what is called a milk scan. This is very similar to the gastric emptying test used in adults, but the radioactive tracer is added to milk instead. It allows the doctors to evaluate whether the baby has reflux and also the rate at which the milk empties through the stomach.

Personal Experience Part 3

I finally got in to see another gastroenterologist. This one was much kinder than the previous one had been and actually seemed to have some interest in my well-being. This contrast in demeanor and approach made an enormous difference for me and gave me a small thread of hope.

This new physician ordered an upper endoscopy and discovered that I had no peristalsis in my upper GI tract. This included both my esophagus and stomach. He didn't look past my stomach because, as he said, he "had seen enough". He prescribed another drug called erythromycin and instructed me to take it 4 times a day, 30 minutes before meals.

I did as I was told, only to discover that erythromycin caused my stomach to cramp painfully every time that I took it. I took it prior to lunch at work one day and found myself doubling over in pain. Needless to say, I did not eat lunch that day, or much of anything for a couple of days until I was certain that the erythromycin was doing more harm than good.

This doctor responded quickly to my concerns with erythromycin. He made an effort to get a new drug, tegaserod (Zelnorm), approved for me to use at a very high dose. It was actually approved to treat constipation, but some small studies had shown that it might help with stomach emptying. I was able to take samples for a couple of months, but it had little impact. Insurance never agreed to pay for it, so I gave up on it. Zelnorm was pulled from the market a couple of years later due to possible risks to the heart.

At this point, my gastroenterologist admitted that he didn't know what else to do for me and referred me to a motility specialist about 1.5 hours away from my house, in San Francisco. This doctor did not have a kindly demeanor, nor did he seem to care about my health. But he was an expert in the field and after waiting months for my first appointment with him, he immediately set about running all of the tests to diagnose me.

He ordered another upper endoscopy to allow him to make his own evaluation. I had my third emptying test, except that this one was 6 hours long, something that he considered the gold standard. I will reiterate here how much I hate tasting those eggs! I don't know that the doctors really understand that something that tastes disgusting to begin with gets to taste bad over and over again for those of us with active regurgitation.

This was also the day that I had my esophageal manometry. This exam lasted for 4 hours during which time they tested a battery of drugs to see how they impacted the movement of my esophagus. Then I was asked to drink Ensure in an effort to evaluate the impact of food on those movements. Some of those medications caused my stomach to contract tightly and cramp up painfully. All I had eaten that day was the food for the emptying test, and I had developed a headache from low sugar and dehydration. I remember begging them to give me some type of intravenous pain medication or at least fluids for what was turning into a pounding headache, but they insisted that all that I could have was a cup of liquid Tylenol.

After a day and a half of testing, this new specialist made an appointment to go over my results. I waited for three hours after the appointment start time before he arrived for what ended up being a 20-minute discussion. He officially diagnosed me with gastroparesis. At that point, this was not news, although it had never been official before. And then he told me that 3 of 5 cases resolve spontaneously within 5 years, and so I should just wait it out and see what happens. Because I had only been sick for 3 years, I was not a candidate for the gastric neurostimulator (much more on this later), nor did he think that there were any other medications worth trying. He gave me a standing prescription for anti-nausea medication and sent me on my way.

The devastation hit immediately. I had gone to this appointment with exceptional hope. This doctor was an expert, he had ordered all of these tests, he held so many promising therapies in his hands – this was my chance. I felt nothing less than utter despair while walking out of his office. This arrogant man had made me wait in his office for 3 hours with no apology and made a cold, calculated decision to not provide me with any treatment options based solely on the timeframe of my illness. There was no regard for my person, my symptoms, or my quality of life.

I still fought for a little while. I called his office and asked for a prescription for domperidone based on my own research. I found a compounding pharmacy to make it and finally obtained a prescription from his office. Unfortunately, it did not help me. I eventually called the office to let them know and ask what, if any, options I might have at this time. I never heard back.

Gastroparesis and Taking Medications

5

"It is what we think we know already that often prevents us from learning."

CLAUDE BERNARD

One might wonder how being a pharmacist really provides much insight into managing gastroparesis. I know that I mulled over that for a while, contemplating how I landed in a branch of the medical profession that did not have much to offer in the way of relief for a person with my condition.

I actually decided that I wanted to be a pharmacist back in high school. I had originally wanted to attend medical school and become a doctor. In fact, I was much more specific than that. I had an underactive thyroid as a child, which very briefly introduced me to one small segment of healthcare and brought about only the most practical of childhood goals – becoming a pediatric endocrinologist. While volunteering at a hospital in high school, it didn't take much time with the physicians that I spoke with to pick up on a major theme – no doctor recommended that I follow in their footsteps. Even though I was wholly susceptible at the time to the youthful pitfall of "But I'm not going to end up where they are!", this still looked like a big, flashing warning light.

Then I met some of the pharmacists in the hospital, who all loved what they did. And I realized that it just so happened that what they did sounded like what I had really wanted out of my super realistic career goal in pediatric endocrinology. I wanted to learn about the way that the molecules in the body interacted with and impacted the body.

It turns out that what originally drew me to pharmacy is still incredibly pertinent to those of us with gastroparesis. It also turns out that having gastroparesis introduces a new layer that must be considered regarding the interactions of molecules with the body. This new layer has two equally important sides:

1. Medications change the way that gastroparesis (and other GI conditions) acts

2. Gastroparesis changes the way that medications work

Every person with gastroparesis will have "ah-ha!" moments as we jump into this topic. But as far as I know, there is no information out there that really examines or evaluates this layer. While it is incredibly important to me to provide highly referenced and evidence-based information, the information that we will discuss in this section, is, by nature, primarily a product of blending my knowledge as a pharmacist into my experience with gastroparesis.

MEDICATIONS IN THE GI TRACT

When we discussed the GI tract earlier in the book (see page 29), it was focused on explaining how the foods that we eat move through the GI tract, and where the nutrients in that food are absorbed. I didn't mention much about how medications fit into that process. But in order to really understand how medications and gastroparesis can interact, we're going to do that now.

Medications are also absorbed from the GI tract, just like the nutrients in the foods that we eat. However, there are some key differences in how and where they are absorbed.

An important point is that medications can be absorbed throughout the GI tract. Absorption can even occur in the mouth, as I mentioned previously regarding orally disintegrating tablets. From there they can be absorbed in the stomach, different portions of the small intestine, and even in the large intestine (colon). There are a number of factors that play into where each medication is absorbed, but we will focus on just two.

1. **The drug itself**

   Each drug is a molecule. The size of that molecule can have a say in which part of the GI tract is able to absorb it. In addition, some molecules respond favorably to acids and some respond favorably to bases. Which environment the molecule likes the most also has a large say in which part of the GI tract is able to absorb it.

2. **The form of the drug**

   The formulation that the drug is provided in makes a huge difference in where the drug is absorbed. In fact, many dosage forms are made for the purpose of forcing a drug to be absorbed in a specific place. You might have heard terms like "enteric-coated" or "extended-release" thrown around. These are often formulations that are made specifically to guide a drug to a certain part of the GI tract for absorption, and we will talk about them more in this chapter.

The drug industry has created all kinds of terms that simply indicate that the absorption of the medication has been altered, such as:

1. Extended-release (XR, ER, XL)
2. Delayed-release (DR)
3. Controlled-release (CR)
4. Sustained-release (SR)
5. Enteric-coated (EC)

Additionally, how the drug is absorbed is very dependent on what is happening around the drug while it is in the GI tract. You are all familiar with drugs that "should be taken with food" or "should be taken on an empty stomach". You might also be aware of some medications that cannot be taken with certain vitamins and minerals (i.e. calcium or iron). Each molecule interacts differently with the GI tract and the environment around it. Some drug molecules bind to vitamins, minerals, or food and this keeps them from being absorbed. Some drug molecules must compete with the nutrients in the food to be absorbed, which reduces the amount of the drug that makes it into the body.

Yet other molecules are absorbed better when they are swimming in fats, leading to increased absorption when taken with fatty foods. There are many scenarios, but environment is quite important for drug absorption.

Now that we've established these general concepts, let's walk quickly through the GI tract again, except this time we will see it from the perspective of a drug.

You'll notice that some of the pieces of the GI tract are missing. That is just because you already know about them and they don't apply here!

MOUTH

Most drugs are swallowed, and so they skip this area entirely. However, some drugs are sucked on, chewed, or placed into the cheek. Medications that are chewed undergo mechanical digestion in the mouth and are then swallowed for processing through the GI tract, just as you would expect with food. Medications that are sucked on might be absorbed in the mouth (i.e. orally disintegrating tablets) or might simply be slowly dissolved and then swallowed for processing through the GI tract. Medications that are placed in the cheek (buccal) are typically absorbed entirely through the mouth.

ESOPHAGUS

The esophagus doesn't really play much of a role outside of carrying the medications down to the stomach. However, I did want to point out that some medications must be taken with a full glass of water, or must be taken while sitting upright. There is a legitimate reason for this guidance that you find on the medication bottle and paperwork – if the medications get stuck in the esophagus on the way down, they can actually start to damage it. Just a friendly note from a pharmacist!

STOMACH

Many medications will be broken down in the stomach. The tablet or capsule might dissolve or disintegrate here, releasing the molecule. For some medications, the acidic environment of the stomach is a great place for absorption, and some molecules will begin to be absorbed right here. That's a quick turnaround time from when you popped the pill! A good example of this rapid absorption in the stomach and quick effect is one of the world's favorite drugs - alcohol.

DUODENUM/JEJUNUM

I am combining these two because for the purposes of medications, we can just knock them out at once. The small intestine is where the large majority of drugs are absorbed. Since this part of the GI tract is built to absorb nutrients, it also happens to be well primed for absorbing medications. Some may be absorbed in the duodenum, some in the jejunum, and some in both. Some drugs are even absorbed in both, plus the stomach. In fact, the way that some "extended-release" and "delayed-release" drugs are made encourages them to be absorbed little by little throughout the GI tract, to allow small doses of the drug to enter the body over time. This can be done in a number of ways, but some of the most common are to use a special coating or a special capsule that dissolves at a very slow rate.

LARGE INTESTINE

There are a small number of drugs that are absorbed in the large intestine. Some of those extended-release and delayed-release drugs will also be absorbed here. Some medications are only absorbed here. I mentioned previously that some of the bacteria in the gut is actually involved in breaking down a small number of drugs (see page 39). That typically happens in the large intestine, and then they are absorbed.

RECTUM

Finally, there are actually medications that are never absorbed from the GI tract. These medications are those that are meant to only have an effect within the GI tract, such as medications for

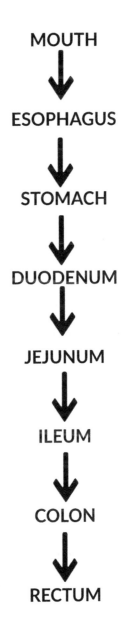

MOUTH

↓

ESOPHAGUS

↓

STOMACH

↓

DUODENUM

↓

JEJUNUM

↓

ILEUM

↓

COLON

↓

RECTUM

constipation or a number of the drugs available to treat ulcerative colitis. In this case, they will pass all the way through, from the mouth to the anus, without ever being absorbed into the rest of the body.

GASTROPARESIS: IMPACTING MEDICATIONS

Now that we've traveled back through the GI tract from the perspective of a medication, we can discuss the extra layer that gastroparesis adds to the picture.

Just as with foods, medications require peristalsis to move them consistently along through the GI tract to their destination. And just as with foods, motility delays will lead to delays in the transit of medications through the GI tract. Another point to consider is that when medications and foods are delayed at the same time, they spend a lot of time hanging out together. When we talked about the symptoms of gastroparesis, we mentioned that there are "downstream effects" of delayed stomach emptying that echo all the way through the GI tract, leading to additional symptoms (see page 46). In the same way, this delay can also lead to impacts for medications throughout the GI tract.

Delays in motility lead to delays in medication absorption. Has anyone ever noticed that it takes longer to see the effect of some drugs than they would like? I know that I was not thrilled when I realized this was happening. This impacts me most when I'm trying to take a pain reliever for a headache or muscle ache. Over-the-counter medications that are taken only when needed for certain situations are the biggest culprits. These are exactly the times when you want the medication to work as quickly as possible!

There's another type of medication that this can be a big problem for - birth control. We will talk about the possible impacts with this class of medications in the second part of the book.

People with gastroparesis also have food in their stomachs for much longer than most people. I know that if I try to eat snacks/meals throughout the day, I will be aware of having food in my stomach for almost the entire day from the moment that I start eating. Thus, it makes it very difficult to obey instructions when they include something like "take on an empty stomach". There are times in the morning when I have an empty stomach, but that is not always the case. And I know, for me, it is rare to have an empty stomach at any point in the day after that.

The traditional guidance for taking a medication on an empty stomach is 1 hour before or 2 hours after eating. You can see how this might be difficult to abide by if you experience a significant delay in emptying.

For medications that need to be taken on an empty stomach, this can be a problem. For medications that cannot be taken with certain vitamins or minerals, this can also be a problem. The medication might bind to something else and be unable to be absorbed. It might have to compete with the nutrients that are around it to be absorbed and be unsuccessful in doing so. It is very important to give your medications the best chance at working by identifying the times that your stomach is most likely to be empty or by avoiding the nutrients that might interact with it.

I mentioned previously that I have an underactive thyroid. This means that I have to take levothyroxine (Synthroid) every day to replace the hormones that my body is not producing on its own. Synthroid is one of those medications that should be taken on an empty stomach and that also interacts with other nutrients, such as calcium. Although I take it in the morning (my best chance at an empty stomach) and try hard to separate it from any dairy products, I haven't been very successful at getting the full effect from that medication. Since I developed gastroparesis, the dose of Synthroid that I have to take has actually doubled. And a few years ago I even had to change to a brand new form of the drug - a gel capsule. It took many years and a lot of frustration and symptoms for me to finally obtain a steady and appropriate level of levothyroxine in my body.

We will talk much more about how to make different drug formulations work more effectively for you later in this section.

Other GI conditions can also have an impact on the way that medications are processed by the body. For instance, those with Crohn's disease in the small intestine experience a lot of inflammation. This inflammation might actually increase the amount of a medication that is absorbed, going beyond what is expected. Although that is not the focus of this book, it is important to realize that any changes to the GI tract can impact the items that are moving through it.

MEDICATIONS: IMPACTING GASTROPARESIS

I mentioned earlier that there are two sides to this coin - medications also have an impact on gastroparesis. This may seem counterintuitive on the surface, but most of those with gastroparesis have likely experienced this multiple times.

There are many situations in which medications that are used to treat one condition can actually cause issues for another condition. Since doctors don't often spend a lot of time focusing on discussing possible side effects, we don't usually think about medications this way. We are more focused on what it will do for the condition that it was prescribed to treat. But in reality, medications can do a lot more than just the one thing that they were intended for. When it comes to the GI tract, this can happen in a number of ways, so we will touch on each of them separately.

1. **Slowing of GI motility**

    Some drugs can actually slow GI motility further. As you can imagine, this could then worsen any gastroparesis symptoms that are already present due to slowed motility. These medications include narcotics, anti-diarrheals (i.e. Immodium), alcohol, and some older antidepressants that are used for a number of different indications, including irritable bowel syndrome and nerve pain (e.g. amitriptyline or nortriptyline).

We will be back to talking about these pesky narcotics before you can turn the page!

2. **Loosening the esophageal sphincter**

    We talked about the esophageal sphincter becoming loose in our discussion of the GI tract, and here we are again (see page 32)! When this sphincter becomes loose, it makes it easier for food to travel back up into the esophagus from the stomach, something that can be uncomfortable and concerning over time. There are actually a number of foods that can cause this to happen, including spicy foods and chocolate. But there are also a lot of medications that are known for this. One of the medication classes that is most associated with this, used for high blood pressure and heart conditions, is calcium channel blockers, such as amlodipine (Norvasc), nifedipine, and felodipine. Other medications that can loosen the sphincter include narcotics, I told you! female hormones, cigarettes and nicotine, and some muscle relaxants known as benzodiazepines (e.g. Valium or Xanax).

3. **Symptom overlap**

This will be different for each person with gastroparesis since each of us typically experiences a different array of symptoms. But when a medication causes a side effect that happens to be a symptom that you already have, this can make it noticeably worse. For instance, if you experience a lot of nausea and constipation and take a medication that can cause nausea and constipation, you may experience a worsening of your symptoms. This is called an "additive effect". Symptoms that are most likely to be affected by this include nausea, vomiting, constipation, diarrhea, bloating, and gas.

4. **"GI upset"**

The terms "GI upset", "GI discomfort", and "gastrointestinal side effects" are used as a blanket to cover all kinds of undefined irritation that medications can cause to the GI tract. If a medication is known to cause GI upset, then there is a chance that those with gastroparesis will be more acutely aware of this change. It can include stomach pain, nausea, vomiting, bloating, diarrhea, loose stools, and more. The positive side here is that there are often ways to prevent GI upset from medications. In fact, one of the most common ways is to take these medications with food. It is always worth inquiring on whether there are ways to minimize these side effects to make these medications more tolerable to take.

We're back to narcotics again! Just to clarify what this group of drugs actually includes, below is a list of the most common ones:

- Hydrocodone (Vicodin, Norco)
- Oxycodone (Oxycontin)
- Hydromorphone (Dilaudid)
- Oxymorphone (Opana)
- Morphine
- Methadone

I want to take a moment to talk about those repeat offenders – narcotics. This class of medications is well known for causing nausea and vomiting. It is also quite well known for causing constipation. In fact, these drugs cause constipation by slowing the motility in the lower GI tract. If you take narcotics for an extended period of time and don't also take something to prevent constipation, this can actually cause some dangerously severe constipation that could require surgery. Considering that narcotics can also loosen the esophageal sphincter, strategies to avoid using narcotics should definitely be considered for the average person with gastroparesis.

It is difficult to provide a complete list of the drugs that can be responsible for all of the concerns that we discussed above. But many of those side effects can actually be found with the packet of information that comes with the medication. It is also helpful to ask your pharmacist about any very specific concerns that you have (such as loosening of the esophageal sphincter), as they will be able to find this information for you in reliable resources that likely require paid access.

You can now take the four general points that we just discussed and apply them to any medication, whether it is listed in this section or not.

The information discussed above is mostly general and conceptual. While this might at first seem overwhelming and difficult to apply, it is actually meant to be of use to you far longer than information referring to specific medications would allow.

You will notice this theme develop as we move along through this book. What you are learning here will be of service to you in finding the appropriate information that you need regarding all of the medications that you might take in the future. There are thousands of drugs already on the market, and that number is growing every year. You are being armed with the right questions to ask of the people who can answer them and with the concepts necessary to understand how a medication might impact you (or what your gastroparesis can do to it). This will allow you to manage your own care no matter what is thrown at you!

For medications, your best resource is always a pharmacist. But it's important to find one that you like and trust, that will be patient and receptive to your concerns.

OTHER WAYS TO TAKE MEDICATIONS

Being aware of how gastroparesis and medications can interact with each other will allow you to look for certain types of information before starting to take a medication. It will also allow you to ask the right questions from the doctor when it is prescribed, and the pharmacist when it is filled. And finally, it will allow you to be more aware of changes that might occur after you have started taking that medication.

But it is also possible for you to try to minimize the impact that gastroparesis can have on some of the medications that you might be taking. I mentioned earlier that it is important to give your medications their best chance at working. This can be possible by abstaining from vitamins or minerals that are known to bind with the medication, or taking the medication at the time of day that you are most likely to have an empty stomach (if that is the environment required for that particular medication).

Another consideration is the possibility of altering the form of the medications that you are taking. This includes crushing tablets, opening capsules, or getting a pharmacy to prepare the medication in liquid form. Other considerations even include getting the medication through a non-oral route. The sheer number of questions that I have gotten about the ways that medications can be altered is one of the ways that I know many people with gastroparesis have the experience of medications sitting in their stomachs indefinitely. So let's talk about it!

One of the ways to try to get a tablet go down easier is to break it up before you even start to swallow it. Some of the approaches to this are to dissolve it in a liquid or crush it with a kitchen instrument.

It is very important to recognize that this is not a good idea for all tablets. For instance, I mentioned earlier that some medications are specifically made to slowly release throughout the GI tract (extended-release and delayed-release products). If the release mechanism is destroyed by crushing the tablet, then the entire dose of that medication will be absorbed at once, which can be dangerous and cause additional side effects or toxicity. Other medications have what is called enteric coating. This coating allows the tablet to pass through the stomach to the small intestine before dissolving. The reason for this may be that the medication can actually harm the stomach tissue, or because the acid in the stomach will deactivate the medication. Eliminating this coating could potentially lead to stomach damage over time or render the medication completely ineffective.

The Do Not Crush List was created by an organization called the Institute for Safe Medication Practices (ISMP). They are dedicated to improving the safety of using medications, both in hospitals and at home.

Luckily, there is a handy list that is updated every year called the Do Not Crush List. This list can be found here: http://www.ismp.org/tools/donot-crush.pdf . Although it is called the Do Not Crush list, this also applies to dissolving the medication in a liquid and swallowing it down. In most cases (although there are some exceptions), dissolving the tablet will have the same impact on the dosage form as crushing it.

You will notice that the right-hand column of this list contains a brief description of why the medication should not be crushed. We have already discussed the majority of those reasons here. Some medications will have other, unique issues with crushing that prevents this from being possible. Having this list and the understanding for why a medication is on it will allow you to ask your pharmacist for possible alternative options. Here are some general considerations:

- Sometimes a medication in the same class as one of the drugs on this list can be crushed or dissolved, and your doctor could potentially prescribe that medication in place of the original prescription.

- Extended-release and delayed-release formulations are often just another form of the original medication, which is immediate-release. Immediate-release medications typically need to be taken more often throughout the day (most commonly two or three times daily). Depending on your symptoms and how your gastroparesis affects you, it is possible that being able to crush the immediate-release formulation three times a day would actually be more tolerable to you than taking the extended-release form once or twice a day. Again, this will depend on each individual and is a personal preference.

If the Do Not Crush list leaves you unable to make your medications more digestible, then that just means it is time to get creative! Press your doctor and pharmacist to come up with new solutions using tips like the ones given here.

CAPSULES

A lot of the information regarding manipulating capsules is actually the same as what we just discussed with tablets. However, capsules need to be opened and have their contents dumped out. Sometimes people will want to dissolve these contents in a liquid or mix them with a soft food. Just as with tablets, this might be fine for some capsules and not for others.

Just as with tablets, capsules are also formulated in various ways. There are immediate-, delayed-, and extended-release formulations. In fact, sometimes the contents of the capsule itself are tiny little versions of delayed-release tablets. In those cases, the contents of the capsule can usually be dumped out, but they cannot be crushed or chewed. This would turn them into immediate-release products, a danger that we discussed with tablets.

The same Do Not Crush list can be referenced for capsules as for tablets. And again, the same reasons are provided in the right-hand column. Just as with tablets, it is possible to consider another drug in the same medication class, or another formulation of the same drug to provide a more tolerable alternative for you.

A pharmacist that you trust is a great resource for evaluating all of your options for alternative formulations of both tablets and capsules when you do run into this dilemma. But now you will be able to take that first step of evaluating whether you can crush or dissolve the medication. And you can also consider what options you might be willing to try, allowing you to enter into that conversation with all of the information that you need to help in improving your care.

LIQUIDS

It can be exciting to discover that a medication is available in a liquid form, as these do tend to go down with the least amount of hassle. However, some people will be able to attest that this is not always the case, particularly if a lot of liquid has to be consumed to get the entire dose of the medication. Many liquids are made with sweeteners or stabilizers that can cause side effects when taken in large quantities. The most common side effects are bloating, cramping, and/or diarrhea. It is pretty easy to see how this can overlap with some existing gastroparesis symptoms.

When a smaller dose is needed, that means a smaller volume is required. When an adult needs a large dose, that means there will be more to drink.

A large volume of liquid is most commonly present when that liquid formulation was actually developed for use in children. Not only do children require smaller doses, but children also usually require a lot of sweeteners and flavoring agents to make it palatable. Sometimes, with over-the-counter medications, it might not be possible to get an 'adult version' of that liquid. For instance, liquid ibuprofen (Advil) only comes in the pediatric formulation. However, acetaminophen (Tylenol) comes in both a pediatric liquid and an adult liquid. The adult liquid is much more concentrated and is a much smaller volume.

Adult liquids also taste worse, but that is never surprising with medications!

Another option that is often tempting is to take your prescription to a compounding pharmacy. Some pharmacies will offer to make a liquid version of any medication that you need. However, this is not always appropriate. For instance, when I was in college I had a compounding pharmacy offer to make a liquid version of my Synthroid for me, to make it easier to take. It wasn't until I was in pharmacy school that I learned that liquid Synthroid is unstable. There was almost no drug present in the liquid that I was taking all of that time. This is true of many medications, so it is very important to ask the compounding pharmacist if there is any data available showing that the medication is stable with the recipe that they are using. If there is, they should be able to provide it to you. If there isn't, you probably caught them quite off guard! Again, when you look out for yourself and your own health, you are much more likely to have a positive outcome.

You can bet that I did exactly this when I found out that my medication was probably unstable. This helped to explain why my thyroid levels were so erratic, and has made me incredibly cautious of trusting suggestions that sound too good to be true when it comes to my health.

There is also a drug formulation that can act as a mix between a liquid and a capsule - gel caps. In this case, a very small amount of concentrated liquid is enclosed in a capsule. The capsule will dissolve in the stomach, releasing the liquid for absorption. This can be beneficial for two reasons - the medication may be absorbed more quickly in this form in comparison to a tablet, and it may be more tolerable in certain situations for those with gastroparesis. A great example of an opportunity to use a gel cap for faster absorption is when buying over-the-counter pain relievers, such as naproxen (Aleve). I mentioned previously that I was also able to take advantage of this for my thyroid medication, so when it exists, it is an option worth considering.

NON-ORAL DOSAGE FORMS

Although not very often, it is possible to get some medications into the body without taking them by mouth. The form that people are probably most familiar with is rectally, through either a suppository or an enema. While this is a highly uncomfortable way to take a medication, it can sometimes be incredibly beneficial in urgent situations.

The other alternate way of getting a medication that people are most familiar with is by having it injected. This can be done into the vein (intravenous or IV), into the muscle (intramuscular or IM), or into the skin (subcutaneous or SC). It is definitely preferable to avoid the use of a needle whenever possible, but there are some products that can be given IM or SC that actually last for a long time. This means that the injection only needs to happen once a week, once a month, or possibly even once every few months. Again, this is typically not a preferred option, but it can be considered when other options have been exhausted and the medication that is needed is available in one of these formulations.

Another option is a medication that can be given topically. Most commonly this is provided in the form of a patch. The patch is formulated in such a way that medication is slowly absorbed through the skin and into the body. There are not very many drugs that are made this way, but in the rare cases when they are, this can be very helpful to those with gastroparesis. Even less common is a drug that is available in a cream that can be absorbed into the body.

Compounding pharmacies and their personalized products are not cheap. Know that these personalized suggestions are not typically based on evidence; always be careful of throwing hard-earned money away.

I feel it is again important to mention compounding pharmacies that will be willing to convert a medication to a topical form. It is difficult to develop a cream that is capable of adequately transferring a medication from the skin to the blood stream. In these cases, the biggest danger is that you will pay a lot of money and not receive any benefit from the medication. Just as you should request information regarding any liquid compounds that are offered to you, you should also ask the pharmacist if the cream is made from a recipe with evidence for topical absorption. You will likely take them by surprise with this question, but you are protecting yourself as both a patient and a consumer.

Various studies have been done to evaluate the use of compounded topical creams meant to treat nausea. The appeal of finding a topical treatment for nausea is clear – you don't have to worry about swallowing it, keeping it down, or throwing it back up. These studies have consistently shown that no medication is absorbed into the body from these creams. But, surprisingly, the same studies have also shown that people seem to have less nausea when they use these creams that provide no actual medication! This speaks strongly to the placebo effect, which we will briefly discuss at a later point in this book.

Finally, to wrap up our discussion of alternative ways to get medications, there are some medications that are available in very unusual forms. For instance, Nuvaring is a birth control that is actually available in the form of a thin ring that is inserted into the vagina once a month. A small number of medications can be administered through a pump that is implanted into the body and then slowly delivers the medication over time. More recently, there has been research into a new type of tablet (yes, this is an oral formulation), the mini-tablet. This allows the administration of a dose of medication in a miniature form compared to what we are currently used to. There are also some other exciting prospects with this formulation, but we will have to wait and see where this idea goes!

There are also studies that have shown that the higher the cost of the placebo, the more likely it is to have an effect. So maybe those high price tags actually have a purpose! But I digress. If you have further interest in the fascinating topic of the placebo effect, I would recommend Placebo: Mind Over Matter in Modern Medicine by Dylan Evans.

Mini-Tablets:

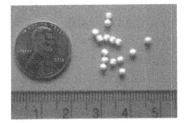

Personal Experience Part 4

I resigned myself to be sick and depressed. It sure didn't seem like anyone cared or had any interest in helping me. Maybe this was just my fate and I should just adjust my expectations and my life around it. I was spinning in hopeless circles and making no improvements whatsoever.

Around this time, my younger sister developed a severe case of colitis. She saw a pediatric gastroenterologist about her condition and really liked her doctor, who took an interest when my mom told her about my case. I was pushing the limits of an age that could be treated by a pediatric physician (I was already 21 and graduated from college), but she agreed to see me anyways. As a side note, my sister's colitis ended up being antibiotic-induced and it self-resolved, which was a relief!

She immediately recognized that I had severe constipation and scheduled me to come into the hospital to have a 'clean-out'. This basically involved administering Golytely (a very large dose of the drug that is found in Miralax) very rapidly through a tube that is placed into the stomach through the nose. This forces intake of the liquid at a rate that is not tolerable for someone with delayed emptying. When I was admitted, the nurse placed the wrong tube down my nose. She used a trauma tube that is meant for patients that need to have their stomachs pumped. It caused me exceptional pain and nausea for 6 hours before my doctor finally stopped over to ask why I was having so many issues and yelled at the nurse the second she discovered the cause.

Once I had been "cleaned out", she was hopeful that my emptying would improve slightly. Unfortunately, it did not. She then prescribed polyethylene glycol (Miralax) to be taken daily to keep me from becoming backed up again and relieve some of my symptoms. I didn't realize at the time that the Miralax was the reason for the increased bloating and gas that I began experiencing because I didn't even think to watch for that as a side effect.

She also performed an upper GI endoscopy and decided that she wanted to try something a little more experimental. She had noticed that my pyloric sphincter was tight and thought that my emptying might be improved by loosening that sphincter. This could be done by injecting Botox into the sphincter muscle in a short procedure. I had this performed twice but experienced no benefits. The doctor had no further ideas for treatment but told me to call if she could be of help in any way.

At this point I was in pharmacy school and had been sick for 5 years. I had no more faith that the medical system could provide me with any help. I was sick of pointless tests and treatments that just made me feel worse. My nutritional status was starting to fail. I had deficiencies in various vitamins. My protein was low. I was losing muscle mass that I have never been able to regain. I had an iron deficiency that was causing me to lose sleep by causing restless leg syndrome. I was exhausted all of the time and struggling to maintain my grades, my job, and any semblance of a life.

The Brain and The Gut 6

"Worry is the stomach's worst poison."

ALFRED NOBEL

At this point we have established a lot of important foundational concepts. We started by discussing the basics of evaluating information and understanding the changes in science. We then moved on to draw a clear picture of the GI tract and the bacteria that inhabit it, using this to explain what gastroparesis is and why it causes the symptoms that it does. We were then able to take this understanding and expand upon it by talking about the ways that medications and our GI tract interact. But we are still missing a discussion regarding an entirely separate organ, and it is not one that we traditionally think of in relation to the GI tract and GI conditions.

The human brain is a powerful thing. It is the most complex brain known to exist on this planet, and it is the most complex organ in the human body. Without it, the body ceases to function. It contains around 86 billion neurons (nerve cells) and trillions of synapses (brain cell connections).

This is that astronomical number that we discussed when we were talking about the number of bacteria in the gut:

1,000,000,000,000

The human nervous system is split into two separate components. The brain is part of what is called the Central Nervous System (CNS), which basically acts as the command center for the body. The CNS also includes the spinal cord and the retina, which is part of the eye. The rest of the nervous system, which acts to connect all of the nerves in the body back to the spinal cord and brain, is called the

Peripheral Nervous System (PNS). This expands out into your hands and arms, feet and legs.

There is another way that the human nervous system is divided up - functionally. This means that the human nervous system actually works in two very different ways in the body.

1. **Somatic**

   These are the functions that we most often associate with the nervous system because it is responsible for coordinating all of our senses and movements. As I type this paragraph, my brain is instructing my somatic nervous system to move my fingers across the keys. And as my fingers are touching the keys that they are pressing, my somatic nervous system sends a signal to my brain where it will be interpreted into a feeling.

   It's those five senses they kept teaching us in school: sight, hearing, touch, smell, and taste.

2. **Autonomic**

   This is the oft forgotten portion of the nervous system because it is responsible for all of the things that our bodies do that we don't have to think about - breathing, regulating blood pressure, and something that we've already discussed, stimulating peristalsis (see page 43). These are involuntary movements. I mentioned previously that gastroparesis can be caused by damage to the vagus nerve (see page 45). Well, guess which part of the nervous system the vagus nerve calls home? Autonomic. But it gets even more specific from there.

THE SECOND BRAIN

The autonomic nervous system has a subdivision known as the enteric nervous system. As would be expected for a part of the autonomic system, it also controls involuntary movements, but it is specific to the movements within the gastrointestinal system. This is the highly specialized portion of the nervous system that is responsible for those coordinated muscle contractions which create peristalsis. In fact, it is so complex that it contains the same number of neurons as the spinal cord. It can even conduct its function completely alone, without any input from the brain!

However, a unique aspect of the enteric nervous system is that even though it functions autonomously, it also communicates regularly with the central nervous system and the brain to add more functionality. For instance, the brain can have a say in how quickly or slowly the food moves through the GI tract. It can also interpret the sight of certain foods into preparatory secretion of specific chemicals in the stomach and intestine. There is a lot more that the brain can do in relation to the enteric nervous system, but for the sake of relevance, we'll stop there.

The complexity of this nervous system is beyond far outside of the scope of this book, so I won't waste any time trying to explain it in great detail. Instead we'll take the basic information that we just covered and move right along into why this is at all important to someone with gastroparesis (I promise that it is!).

The enteric nervous system has earned the special distinction of being called the Second Brain. This is due to the complexity that we already discussed, and the large number of neurons that it contains. It was not until recently that research started to unravel some of the additional functions that this second brain and all of its neural activity may actually be involved in. From this point on, I'm going to do us a favor and simply refer to "the gut" - the combination of the enteric nervous system and the GI tract.

BRAIN-GUT AXIS

The brain and the gut have what has been shown to be two-way communication. That means that the brain can have an influence on what is happening in the gut and the gut can have an influence on what is happening in the brain. This communication stream has been referred to as the brain-gut axis. In fact, this axis has actually been demonstrated to connect the emotional centers of the brain with the gastrointestinal system.

This has some very clear implications to anyone that has or has had a GI condition. Have you ever noticed that stress triggers a worsening of symptoms? That challenges in life seem to compound on each other by adding challenges from gastroparesis as well? Or that focusing on your symptoms negatively affects your mood and psyche? It turns out that this is not in your head and that there is a very real correlation between what your brain is experiencing in the rest of your life and what your GI tract is experiencing from your gastroparesis. We will get into more discussion about this connection in just a bit.

The brain-gut axis is basically a neural and endocrine highway from our minds to our guts. It is surprising how much one can directly influence the other, although limitations to its capabilities do exist.

A very interesting and somewhat unexpected discovery in recent years is the surprising importance of the bacteria in the gut to this communication axis. As we discussed previously, there are thousands of bacterial species in the gut, each with their own unique function and role that we, for the most part, have yet to fully understand (see page 36). Recent research has indicated that these same bacteria are also responsible for sending signals to the enteric nervous system regarding the state of the GI tract in response to the medications and foods to which they are exposed. This is one of those evolving fields of science where we don't have very much confirmed information yet (see page 23). Validating the early discoveries and what we think we know in this field will take years, and any sensational news releases should be considered skeptically until more information is available.

GASTROPARESIS: THE CHICKEN OR THE EGG?

We have established that there is an undeniable two-way connection between our brains and our guts that goes so far as to actually impact our emotions and moods. But do we know if one of those connections is stronger? Or if we can tell which one is pushing harder at any given time and overriding the other? Is our gastroparesis bringing us down, or are we making our gastroparesis symptoms worse?

Technically the axis is called both the brain-gut axis and the gut-brain axis, changing to indicate which direction the signal is moving. But we're not always entirely clear on which direction that is.

When an undesirable mental state occurs for those with gastroparesis, it may be viewed from different perspectives depending on what their lives were like prior to the diagnosis. For instance, people that considered their lives generally happy and balanced prior to developing symptoms may blame the gastroparesis for any current depression or anxiety. This is a reasonable conclusion, considering the social isolation and sudden changes in lifestyle that often come with developing this condition. Studies even exist showing that depression and anxiety occur often in those with gastroparesis and other GI conditions, and that this causation can go in both directions.

For those that dealt with depression or anxiety prior to the development of gastroparesis symptoms, they might note that their mental state remains the same. Or they may see a very real connection between their GI symptom severity and their mental state as it fluctuates. There is evidence to support the concept that those with depression or anxiety may be predisposed to developing certain GI conditions. And it is very accepted that certain psychiatric medications are capable of treating some GI disorders and symptoms, something that we will discuss in more detail in the second half of this book.

The accurate explanation for any situation will depend completely on the personal factors involved and will always vary by the individual. Let's take a look at some of the studies that validate the existence and reality of these considerations.

Most studies that look at this two-way communication in people with GI conditions are not conducted in those with gastroparesis. But one of the largest and most valid studies that has been conducted evaluated people with IBS, GERD and IBD. In this study, they sent out a survey that asked questions about mood and psychological state to a random group of people. Of the 1,000 respondents, 376 had one of these GI conditions.

PROMISING

Twelve years later, they sent out the same survey again, and found that while some conditions had resolved in that time frame, others had developed a GI condition, leaving the total number of people with GI conditions about the same.

- They found that a high level of anxiety at baseline led to a higher chance of developing IBD. A higher level of depression at baseline led to a higher chance of developing GERD.

- They also found that developing these GI conditions increased the chance that someone could develop anxiety or depression.

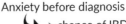

RESULTS:

Depression before diagnosis
↘ > chance of GERD

Anxiety before diagnosis
↘ > chance of IBD

Having a GI condition
↘ > chance of anxiety or depression

A study that was conducted specifically in those with gastroparesis was a little bit different and not as robust. In this study, depression and anxiety surveys were obtained from 300 people with gastroparesis in an effort to correlate these psychological conditions to the severity of gastroparesis symptoms.

 PROMISING

- What they found was that depression and anxiety did appear to worsen as the severity of the gastroparesis increased. Specifically, the worsened symptoms included nausea, vomiting, bloating, and feeling full after eating.

Symptom-Psych Correlation:

Nausea
Vomiting 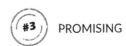 Depression
Bloating Anxiety
Feeling Full

- This indicates that the severity of the psychological condition worsened alongside the severity of certain gastroparesis symptoms. This was not associated with the rate of gastric emptying or with what caused the gastroparesis in the first place.

Unfortunately, this study does not provide any information on which direction this negative message is moving along the brain-gut axis. But it does provide an indicator that either condition can likely cause a worsening in the other.

Again, not all of these were able to determine the cause versus the effect. But the association is very real.

There are a number of additional studies that have looked at conditions other than gastroparesis and established a correlation between psychological state and GI disease severity. There are also some other conversations that have been ongoing regarding the consideration of psychological state in the treatment of gastroparesis and other GI conditions. This information is referenced, but for the sake of brevity, I won't discuss these very similar findings. The studies that we have already looked at thus far provide interesting points for contemplation.

It does appear that GI conditions and psychological conditions can have an impact on each other. It appears that the GI condition may be the chicken or the egg, depending on the specific situation. But it is also important to recognize that the correlation between these two factors actually provides a huge opportunity for us to make an impact on our own situations.

GASTROPARESIS AND PSYCHOLOGICAL STATE

In order to discuss the opportunities that this correlation can represent for our health, I think it's very important to acknowledge and address the impact that gastroparesis can have on our psychological states. My goal here is not to focus on the negative aspects of our lives. Rather, I want to recognize and validate what many of us have and continue to experience so that we can hold an honest conversation about the ways in which we are in control of certain aspects of our quality of life.

You have been following along with my personal experience throughout the book thus far and have likely seen that my journey with gastroparesis has had many lows and disappointments. While it was difficult for me to relive those points in my life, I made an effort to be open and honest about how I felt during those times, including all of the depression and anger they involved. It can be incredibly reassuring and helpful to know that your thoughts and feelings throughout this process are shared by others. I know that as I received emails from readers with gastroparesis, they expressed very similar experiences and emotions. This encouraged me to push forward in my own efforts to improve my quality of life and that of others around me.

While finding others to empathize with is very important, it is also important to keep a positive goal in mind. This positive goal can make the difference between bringing each other down instead of lifting each other up with encouragement.

A LOSS OF SOCIAL EATING

An article that discusses these feelings very well is "A loss of social eating: the experience of individuals living with gastroparesis". This title stood out to me when I first read it. Over the time that it took me to come to terms with the permanence of my condition, I had felt a loss. I could attribute this loss to various areas of my life, but one of the most tangible was the social loss that I incurred. We live in a food-centric culture in which many of our social events and gatherings are based around food. Besides already feeling unwell and less inclined to interact with others, the introduction of food to these interactions can make them even more difficult to face.

I would not refer to this as a scientific study, and I will not rate it on our evidence scale. This article represented an exercise in empathy and an effort on the part of the medical community to obtain a better understanding for the impact that gastroparesis can have on quality of life, as well as the implications this may have for treatment.

Quoted excerpt from A Loss of Social Eating:

"When it comes to eating out, no. I just couldn't. I think that that in itself sometimes is a nightmare because you want to go out and it's like, friends birthdays and that, ... because we were quite close with the neighbours and we used to go out. But I just won't now. I think it's when I eat at home and I need to be sick, I know I am in a safe environment. I've got somewhere to run to quite quickly, but I think it's the thought when you are out, cause like, [sucks breath in through her teeth] Ooh, I could vomit any time."

Nine people with gastroparesis were interviewed for this study, providing in-depth accounts of their experiences, both in relation to symptoms and the social and psychological impact of their diagnosis. Many of those interviewed divided the people in their lives into the grouping of those that understood and those that did not. Many also attributed significant stress and anxiety to interacting with those that did not, and the limitations that it placed on their ability to have regular social interactions and activities. Many voiced the recurring struggles between eating to appease the people around them and not eating to avoid the risk of developing symptoms in front of others.

Many interviewees commented on concerns about being able to control their nausea and vomiting in public. Others mentioned concerns associated with not being able to try foods with others, or "walk down the street snacking" in the way that they were accustomed to. Every person has developed their own habits and rituals associated with eating in a social setting, and these can be significantly disrupted with the development of gastroparesis. In fact, this article even touched on something else entirely – an ingrained human need to participate in the act of eating. Even when food is not needed for nutritional reasons (i.e. for those receiving tube feeds), people still crave the act of eating and chewing on food.

Quoted excerpt from A Loss of Social Eating:

"They felt accused of fabrication if no physical causes were found: 'It's not in my head, I'm not lying'. 'It's not something I've brought on myself to be ill'."

There was also mention of the disbelief they have encountered from physicians and family members. This involved the implication or overt statement that the symptoms must be all in their heads or something that they are doing to themselves. Many of the people interviewed described new insecurities and an experience of developing a new identity in relation to the social structure around them.

People with gastroparesis can empathize with these feelings and experiences and many more at that. Many of us battle the desire to collapse into ourselves on some days and avoid other human beings entirely. Many of us choose to make personal sacrifices on a regular basis to make the people around us happy. I can only imagine the other examples that many of you could add. Whether this has been a recent diagnosis or something that has been managed for years, the social pressures and concerns never go away. However, as time goes on and we become more familiar with our symptoms, triggers, and needs, we have the opportunity to embrace this experience and become veterans in what to expect and how to navigate those difficult situations and concerns.

CHANGING PERSPECTIVES

The study that we have been discussing did not stop at assessing the psychological impact that gastroparesis had on the individuals in the interviews. It also assessed the psychological impact that their choices in handling this condition had made on them. In this study and outside of it, the approach to this type of life change is typically handled in three general ways:

A. This diagnosis I have received is difficult, frustrating, and unfair. I will dedicate all of my energies to finding a way to get rid of it so that I can get my life back to normal.

B. I am my disease and I need to give in to the changes that it demands of me. My life will never be the same and I have to just admit that my quality of life will never be good again.

C. This condition is not who I am, it is simply another difficulty that I must face in life. I am lucky to not be in a worse situation (i.e. diagnosed with cancer or terminally ill) and I should do everything I can to discover the ways that I can improve my quality of life as much as possible.

These perspectives could be abbreviated as follows:

A. Denial
B. Resigned Acceptance
C. Determined Acceptance

These will correlate both with where we are in our journeys and also with our emotional states in relation to other aspects of our lives.

While these are the three general approaches that a person can take, many people may fall somewhere in between these, some will fall into all of these throughout their journeys, and some will have very unique experiences. For instance, many of us will experience A immediately after diagnosis, and it will last for different lengths of time depending on each person. I know that I languished in this approach for longer than I probably should have.

Sometimes, after progressing past A, we may move into B or right along into C. We could even progress very far forward with approach C, only to find ourselves regressing into B during difficult times. I know that I have done exactly that, and it is very important to stress the normalcy of these emotional cycles and struggles over time. Just as someone without gastroparesis cannot manage to be positive at all times, neither can someone with gastroparesis. Every person enters periods of depression and self-doubt in their lives and the additional introduction of gastroparesis to this cycle can very practicably exacerbate these times of struggle.

Quoted excerpt from A Loss of Social Eating:

"So you could completely fall into what is happening and you could go down like to, I don't know, I call it the depression route. So, you know, you are very like, you are very like ... engrossed in like what's happening, like the illnesses, they sort of eat you up?"

In the Loss of Social Eating article, there were interviewees who considered themselves to be defined by their disease, as well as some that considered themselves to be separate from their condition. Those that were defined by their disease found themselves isolated and removed from social life and interactions, dependent on others to care for their needs consistently. They had resigned themselves to being a "gastroparesis patient", or someone with poor quality of life that could not be improved.

Quoted excerpt from A Loss of Social Eating:

"It makes you feel more a part of life. If you're in with a chance of doing something and keeping yourself positive, for me it's having goals. I will go out on my bike, I will go and do this, or go and do that. And even when I'm sick I will say to myself, my goal is to get out of bed and sit downstairs. To every day person that may not seem much, but when you feel really ill and feel absolutely awful, to manage to get out of bed and sit down stairs, even if you are still being sick, is quite a big thing. It just proves that I can do it."

However, there were a larger number of interviewees that had the opposite viewpoint. They considered themselves lucky to not be in a worse situation. They went out of their way to find social activities that did not involve food in order to keep themselves from becoming isolated. Many of them made a strong effort to stay busy, to focus on other aspects of life, and to downplay their condition to themselves and those around them.

One of the very important points that was made in this article was that the decision to move forward with life despite having gastroparesis was not possible until each person had accepted their condition as permanent. Once they had moved past the hope of having it cured or finding a perfect treatment, they were able to focus on how to coordinate their lives around this new change and to appreciate the things that they were still lucky to have.

Quoted excerpt from A Loss of Social Eating:

"You almost overcompensate in terms of what you will do in a day because I'm not going to be defeated by this."

I do not want to turn this section or this book into a discussion of coping techniques. There are others much more knowledgeable and educated in such endeavors that should be turned to for information on this topic. But I do want to give deserved recognition to the very important role that each of us plays in managing our symptoms, courtesy of that communication highway between our first and second brains - the brain-gut axis.

Regardless of whether or not we know which direction the communication is going on any given day or which brain is responsible for how we are feeling during a certain period in our lives, we should never ignore the fact that we have the power to choose the communication that goes in one of those directions.

Now, I will qualify my use of the word 'power' in that statement. I recognize the involuntary and debilitating impact that true mental health issues can have on a person and the difficulty that any person, with or without gastroparesis, can have in navigating their way through them. I am in no way minimizing the reality of mental health issues. I am instead strongly encouraging their recognition and appropriate treatment in order to allow each person to maximize their quality of life. For those that genuinely struggle with clinical anxiety or depression, counseling can be an essential tool in navigating through these illnesses. For those that are struggling acutely or are not benefiting from counseling or coping techniques alone, medications are another possible option. I am not a mental health professional, and will refrain from making treatment suggestions for diagnosed mental health issues. But should a reader have any such concerns, I encourage you to push past the feared stigma that comes with these types of discussions and consult the appropriate professionals to help you in your journey.

If you have health insurance, never hesitate to use it to its full capacity and explore all of your available options.

If you are not sure if seeing a counselor or psychologist is right for you, schedule a consultation! They are typically covered with reasonably low copays.

For those that fall victim to the more typical ups and downs that come with the challenges of life and the social and dietary challenges of gastroparesis, we have an important opportunity to dramatically improve our symptoms. As I said, I am by no means an expert in coping strategies! All that I can provide are some core ideas to consider, my own experience, and the reassurance that many with gastroparesis do find their own individual approaches to improving their quality of life.

- Place focus on the positive aspects of life, including the recognition that while not ideal, a life with gastroparesis is better than other challenges that could be faced

- Develop a support network that is filled with people that understand your condition and encourage you in your journey

  - This network does not need to be large – a small handful of understanding people can work wonders in counteracting the negativity of a much larger crowd

- Focus on the ways that you can improve your own quality of life through the simple changes, such as diet management, physical activity, and enjoyable hobbies

- Reduce your day-to-day and chronic stress as much as possible and recognize the situations and events that might exacerbate it, altering your coping and eating strategies accordingly

- Keep yourself busy and distracted, even on the difficult days, in order to prevent the downhill slide of dwelling on your symptoms and the negative aspects of your diagnosis

This is an incredible video that showcases the importance of empathy and the need to consider invisible problems.

https://youtu.be/cDDWvj_q-o8

- Learn from the lack of empathy that you have experienced as someone with an invisible condition by extending empathy to difficult people through the recognition that they might also be experiencing difficulties of which you are not aware

Some of these may come naturally to you or you may have already incorporated many of these into your management strategy. But a combination of the above and the addition of your own unique ideas and flavor will give you the strength and ability to use the brain-gut axis to your advantage in your journey to improving your health and quality of life.

Never forget that mood shifts and setbacks are normal, and never place unrealistic expectations on yourself to maintain a certain outlook or appearance at all times. Every person has ups and downs, every person hits roadblocks and difficulties in their lives, and every person must go through the emotional cycle of recognizing, accepting, addressing, and managing these changes. Blaming yourself for experiencing a setback or having a negative thought will only increase your stress level and make it more difficult to manage your symptoms. We are all human and what matters is that the sum of our energy and focus is toward the improvement of our own lives and the lives of others.

Personal Experience Part 5

I was continuing to lose weight and was still deficient in many nutrients. I was also losing the energy to perform basic tasks and for the first time in my life, was frightened that I might not have the energy to work or keep my grades where I wanted them to be in graduate school. After about a year of becoming less healthy and more depressed about my situation, I finally realized that I had no one to turn to but myself. No doctors that I had seen had any more to offer me. No dieticians seemed to have any idea what I needed. My family and friends might try to be helpful, but the typical suggestions of eating healthy foods that only came up and never went down did more harm than good.

I began to really focus closely on my diet. What were the foods that made me the sickest? What were the foods that gave me the smallest number of problems? What were the foods that my body seemed to crave when I wasn't feeling well or that I turned to when I wasn't feeling well ("comfort foods")? I began eliminating problem foods from my diet, regardless of how much I loved them. I began trying to increase the variety of the items that went down well or that didn't cause me many issues. I tried eating certain foods at only certain times to lessen the symptoms that they caused or the discomfort of having to deal with them (i.e. before or during a large social gathering, before or during a stressful event at work or school, etc).

I think it's really important for me to say here that I am not sure I would have been as successful in my diet modifications at any previous point in my struggle with gastroparesis. I am a fighter, and when I was fighting to have gastroparesis "fixed" or ameliorated, that was my only focus. It was not until I admitted defeat in that pursuit that I really gathered the energy and motivation necessary to make drastic lifestyle changes. Cutting out an enormous number of foods that I loved only became possible when I was willing to admit that this was the only way to get better. Overhauling my intake, including what I ate and when and how I ate it, was only possible through the understanding that this was my sole option, and the only person that I could rely on to feel better was myself.

I also began experimenting with new options to combat one of my biggest symptoms, constipation. I was taking Miralax, but it was causing an excessive amount of bloating and gas. So I had replaced one problem with two others. And I can't say that the new ones were more pleasant!

Over time, my water intake had reduced dramatically due to my constant regurgitation that I had mentioned before. I had discovered that carbonated beverages did something strange in my stomach, turning into more of a thick sludge that did not shoot back up my throat uncontrollably. So, naturally, I had developed a soda addiction. This was not a soda addiction in the traditional sense. I was simply addicted to the carbonation, and soda was the easiest and best tasting way to obtain it because no matter how much I wanted to, I could not stand the taste of plain carbonated water! I realized that I needed to get creative. I had tried some carbonated juices and liked the concept. But juices are incredibly high in sugar, so they are not a sustainable way to obtain all of one's fluids. I began to dilute juice with carbonated water, diluting it further every day to accustom myself to the taste. Pretty soon I was able to drink glasses of water that had only negligible quantities of juice in them to mask the flavor of the carbonated water. And just like that, my constipation all but disappeared. I was free from Miralax and the extensive bloating and gas it caused. This was an emotionally liberating moment in my gastroparesis journey.

When I began to feel incrementally better from the diet changes, I attempted to address another dangerous rut that I had fallen into - lack of exercise. I had always been an incredibly active child and teenager - ballet, tap dance, rollerblading, hiking, you name it. However, when gastroparesis really took its toll, I began to withdraw from those activities. It was difficult to move around and exert myself when I felt full, nauseated, or dizzy most of the time. I was also worried about my ability to perform those activities without having a shaking attack or severe nausea.

That's when I discovered walking. Walking is an incredibly low impact form of exercise that doesn't pressure my stomach as much as other forms or require an enormous amount of exertion. It could also be easily stopped and restarted if symptoms required. While ballet and tap dance were out of the question, I had no excuse not to walk. And I soon discovered that walking was actually incredibly therapeutic. Getting that exercise and fresh air made a huge difference to my psyche, which in turn made a huge difference for my symptoms. Biking is another great, low impact activity. I have enjoyed my share of bike rides, but never fell in love with it in the way that I know many others have. Regardless, I had found my way back in to physical activity, and made an effort to walk a good distance daily.

Additional GI Considerations

7

"People make too much of facts. Also people make too much of gut feelings. Gut feelings probably mean food poisoning."

BRIAN DOYLE

We have established a strong understanding for the function of the GI tract and the ways that gastroparesis can disrupt this function. It is also important for us to understand the number of other GI conditions that can cause very similar symptoms, as there are cases in which these conditions occur alongside gastroparesis. When this happens, the best symptom management can only be obtained by correctly identifying the additional condition and incorporating its appropriate treatment and management into your gastroparesis management plan.

We will cover each of the major GI diseases that can occur in addition to gastroparesis, what their common symptoms are, and how they can be diagnosed. We will also discuss some of the issues that can occur from changes to the bacteria of the gut and from sensitivities to certain dietary ingredients. Finally, when confronted with the possibility of having multiple conditions and diagnoses, it is important to consider each concern systematically and manage your options responsibly and knowledgeably. We will discuss how to do exactly that with all of the information presented in this section.

GASTROESOPHAGEAL REFLUX DISEASE (GERD)

GERD is a common condition, particularly as people age, and can very often occur alongside gastroparesis. I am including it here simply so that we can have a clear understanding for what is meant when GERD is discussed – the flow of stomach acid or stomach contents back into the esophagus. Just as the regurgitation and vomiting that often occurs with gastroparesis likely indicates a malfunction of the esophageal sphincter (see page 32), so does the presence of GERD. In this case, however, the movement of stomach contents is a passive and non-forceful transfer into the esophagus or throat, but not the mouth. This simple backward movement of the stomach acid can lead to burning, chest pain, cough, hoarseness, and sore throat.

This condition can often be confused with indigestion. Indigestion is the direct result of eating a specific item that is disagreeable to your stomach. In contrast, GERD is a persistent condition that may become worse when certain foods are consumed, but it is consistently present. The treatment for GERD typically involves the use of acid reducing medications and/or elimination of the most offending foods from the diet. It can also be beneficial to avoid foods and medications that loosen the esophageal sphincter (see page 60). We will have a more in-depth discussion regarding acid reflux and its treatment options later in the book.

Indigestion: Pain or discomfort in the stomach associated with difficulty in digesting specific foods.

GERD: A chronic digestive disease that occurs when stomach acid, or occasionally stomach contents, flows back into the esophagus.

IRRITABLE BOWEL SYNDROME (IBS)

IBS is a functional disorder, meaning that it causes changes in the way that the GI tract works, but without causing any apparent damage to the tissue of the GI tract. This is a relatively common condition, with somewhere between 5-20% of people across the world having it in some form and severity. The presentation of IBS runs a strange gamut for each individual person and may have a dominant symptom of diarrhea, constipation, or, for some people, a mixture of both.

IBS is a condition that is currently only diagnosable by symptom presentation. There is no official test that allows a doctor to definitively identify the presence of IBS. The tool used for this diagnosis is called the Rome III Criteria and requires someone to have at least two of the following:

1. Symptoms are relieved by going to the bathroom

2. Recognized changes were associated with a difference in stool frequency

3. Recognized changes were associated with a difference in stool appearance

It is important to distinguish between gastroparesis and possible IBS. One way to do this is to consider when the symptoms appeared. For instance, it is unlikely that both would have shown up at the same exact time.

Other indicators that IBS may be present can include excessive straining or urgency when stooling, many and frequent trips to the bathroom, and a feeling of bloating. There is no doubt that some of these symptoms show up for people with gastroparesis at times, including that bloated feeling, or a fluctuation between diarrhea and constipation. However, those with IBS experience these specific symptoms very consistently, to the point that they can lead to a notable reduction in quality of life.

If you feel that this description represents what you have been experiencing for at least three months on a regular basis, then you should speak with your doctor about the possibility that you have a form of IBS, be it mild to severe. Of all GI conditions, IBS severity has the strongest association with mental state and stress and anxiety levels. It is also often connected to the consumption of specific foods, and many of those with IBS choose to attempt various restrictive diets in an effort to alleviate symptoms. Thus, the treatments for IBS may include a combination of stress management, dietary changes, and medications.

INFLAMMATORY BOWEL DISEASE (IBD)

IBD is a condition that actually results in damage to the GI tract. In fact, IBD has been described as a digestive tract on fire, and the inflammation associated with this fire can lead to pain, diarrhea, bleeding, and weight loss. IBD can be localized to only one small area of the GI tract or spread throughout its entirety; it can produce tolerable levels of discomfort or be so damaging that sections of intestine must be surgically removed.

Two distinctive diagnoses fall under the umbrella of IBD:

1. The first is commonly known as colitis and involves inflammation that is limited to the colon (see page 39). Some of you may have heard of ulcerative colitis, which is the type of colitis that is caused by the body attacking its own colon. Other forms of colitis include those caused by bacterial or viral infections. It presents as diarrhea, cramping and pain, bleeding or bloody stools, fever, fatigue, and a constant urge to go.

2. The other distinctive form of IBD is Crohn's Disease, which involves inflammation as a result of the body attacking the GI tract. This can occur anywhere along the GI tract, although it is most commonly found in the intestine. The symptoms seen with Crohn's can be very similar to those with colitis, except that there is typically more pain and less blood.

Technically, Crohn's disease could have an impact anywhere from the mouth to the anus but is most commonly in the intestine. Inflammation only in the colon would be considered colitis. This means that intestinal Crohn's disease occurs either in the small intestine or throughout the entire intestine, both large and small.

Unlike IBS, IBD can be directly diagnosed through tests, including blood draws, imaging, and biopsy of the GI tract through endoscopy or colonoscopy. Diet must be closely managed because the damage to the intestine that occurs with inflammation can actually lead to poor absorption of the nutrients found in food. A number of people with IBD appear to also develop some form of IBS, possibly from the residual damage to the intestine or to a change in the makeup of the bacteria in the gut. There is a

We discussed endoscopy under the tests used to diagnose gastroparesis. It entails placing a camera through the mouth and into the upper GI tract. A colonoscopy is the same process but in reverse - a camera is placed through the rectum and into the lower GI tract.

growing arsenal of medications available to help in the management of both colitis and Crohn's disease.

The symptoms of IBD are often quite distinctive and persistent. In fact, a primary indicator that testing should be sought out includes the presence of diarrhea for at least 6 weeks accompanied by weight loss. If you feel that you are manifesting these symptoms on a consistent basis in addition to what you are experiencing from your gastroparesis, it is worthwhile to ask your doctor about the likelihood that you may have one of these conditions and, if warranted, order the appropriate tests.

CELIAC DISEASE

Celiac disease, for all of the attention it has received lately, only occurs in ~1% of the population. Even with all of the increased focus on gluten and testing, this rate has stayed the same.

Celiac disease has received significant media coverage in recent years due to the focus of the national attention on a specific food component – gluten. It is incredibly important to understand the difference between diagnosed celiac disease and any type of perceived gluten sensitivity.

Celiac disease is another condition in which the body attacks its own intestine, leading to extensive damage. The unique aspect of this condition is that the body is actually developing a response to gluten. When gluten is consumed and discovered in the intestine by the body, this leads to an attack on the intestinal tissue. These attacks are so persistent and severe that they begin to render the intestine incapable of absorbing nutrients.

The primary GI symptoms of celiac disease are diarrhea, cramps, bloating, lactose intolerance, increased reflux, and weight loss. Additional likely findings include vitamin and mineral deficiencies, anemia (low iron in the blood), fatigue, and osteoporosis (often related to low calcium in the blood). There is a clear potential for overlap between the symptoms of Celiac and those of gastroparesis. However, in most cases, the extent to which these symptoms occur with Celiac would be considered very extreme for gastroparesis alone.

The reaction to gluten that occurs with Celiac Disease appears to also cause issues in other parts of the body. Those with Celiac may experience issues with the peripheral nervous system, be at increased risk for other conditions in which the body attacks itself (autoimmune diseases), and be at an increased risk for certain types of cancer. It is clear that a firm diagnosis of the presence or absence of celiac disease is incredibly important for self-care, awareness, and access to appropriate medical care and monitoring. While the only existing treatment for this condition is the complete and permanent removal of gluten from the diet, proper monitoring goes beyond this dietary change. The receipt of an accurate diagnosis should not be taken lightly.

It might be helpful at this time to push past the marketing and gain a clearer understanding for what gluten actually is. Gluten is one of the proteins found in wheat. There are proteins that are similar in structure to gluten that can also be found in rye and barley. However, no other naturally occurring substances should contain gluten. Thus, any other base for a product (such as corn, soy, rice, nuts, or dairy) is, by nature, gluten-free. Many companies have hopped into the gluten-free market by simply raising their prices and labeling their products as gluten-free even though they always have been, such as corn chips, peanut butter, and cheese.

Celiac can be quickly diagnosed with a blood test that looks for the antibodies that are being produced by the body to attack gluten. I am going to make an important point right now that you will see me repeat many times before this section is over – **you cannot be tested for Celiac disease unless you are currently eating gluten**. If these tests are positive, most doctors will want to follow up with an endoscopy in order to confirm the presence of damage to the intestine and also to understand how severe it has become.

If you have already implemented a gluten-free diet in an effort to alter your symptoms, you CANNOT be tested for Celiac disease. You would be required to reintroduce gluten to your diet in order to receive a diagnosis.

To ensure that you are receiving the proper care and advice, seek a definitive medical diagnosis of this condition prior to attempting to self-treat, which may limit your access to the best care and knowledge.

If you are concerned that the information covered here has described your symptoms, absolutely speak with your doctor about this possibility. Please have this discussion and the ensuing tests prior to deciding to experimentally remove gluten from your diet.

DIETARY DISRUPTIONS OF THE GUT

LACTOSE INTOLERANCE

This is a well-known condition that I am only including here to ensure that it is clearly understood in comparison to other dietary disruptions. Lactose intolerance is actually quite common, impacting as many as 65% of adults to different degrees. It occurs because the body is lacking lactase, the enzyme responsible for digesting lactose, the sugar found in milk products.

When lactase is missing, the bacteria in the gut begin to process the lactose sugars found in the milk products that you consume (see page 36). Unfortunately, these bacteria produce byproducts that can cause bloating, gas, and diarrhea. Each person will experience these symptoms to a different extent with different items. For instance, some people that can't tolerate milk can easily tolerate yogurt. Elimination of offending dairy products is the easiest treatment for this condition, made even easier today with the many alternative milk products that are now available. There is also a unique treatment option - the lactase enzyme can actually be taken as a tablet when someone plans to eat dairy-heavy products such as ice cream and cheese.

The popular brand name for this product is Lact-Aid and it can be found on any drugstore shelf. It should be taken immediately prior to eating the items that are likely to cause issues.

SMALL INTESTINAL BACTERIAL OVERGROWTH (SIBO)

We briefly mentioned this condition in our overview of the GI tract and the bacteria that live within it. We know that this is a situation in which the bacteria that reside in the large intestine begin to migrate in the wrong direction and up to the small intestine (see page 39). You will remember from our discussion that the small intestine is home to only a limited number and type of bacteria. As with any other bacteria in or on our bodies, when colonic bacteria begin to migrate to unusual places, the GI tract is not always ready to handle this change (see page 36).

Those with gastroparesis may actually be at increased risk for developing this condition due to our stunted GI motility. Peristalsis is responsible for keeping everything in the GI tract moving in one direction. If this muscle movement is limited or absent, then bacteria become more easily able to move in the wrong direction. It is important to recognize that this increased risk does not mean that everyone with gastroparesis will develop SIBO. Nor does it mean that otherwise healthy people will not be at risk for developing this condition. In fact, the use of medications that slow down intestinal motility, like narcotics (see page 62), can place healthy people at an even higher risk of developing SIBO. Acid reducers can also increase the risk of developing this condition.

Unfortunately, many of the common symptoms of SIBO directly overlap with gastroparesis symptoms. These include gas, bloating, diarrhea, constipation, and pain. Sometimes, in the case of very extensive migration of bacteria, damage to the intestine can occur, leading to vitamin and mineral deficiencies as well as weight loss due to reduced nutrient absorption.

SIBO diagnosis and treatment is still a new science undergoing research, but SIBO can usually be diagnosed with a breath test. This is an interesting testing mechanism because it does not require any type of invasive procedure, such as endoscopy. Instead, you will simply be asked to drink a specific liquid, and a device will then monitor the quantity and type of molecules that you breathe out. These molecules are produced when the bacteria in your intestine process the liquid that you

H. pylori may also sometimes be diagnosed with a breath test.

We will also discuss other conditions which can be diagnosed via breath test. These tests are becoming more common and more reliable as we begin to better understand the bacteria in our guts.

just consumed. Different types of bacteria produce different byproducts, so this test allows a doctor to identify which bacteria, if any, appear to be present in the small intestine. If SIBO is diagnosed, it may be treated with antibiotics that only work within the GI tract and are not absorbed into the body.

CARBOHYDRATE INTOLERANCE

Most sugars (carbohydrates) are easily broken down by the GI tract of the typical person. However, some people do not digest these sugars completely. When this happens, they are then processed by the bacteria in the large intestine, leading to the production of extra gas and liquid. This can cause bloating, constipation, and/or diarrhea. The short-chain, rapidly fermentable carbohydrates that have been most commonly associated with this intolerance are the components of a newer and popular acronym: FODMAPs.

Fermentable
Oligosaccharides
Disaccharides
Monosaccharides
Polyols

These terms probably don't mean anything to most people (I personally do not typically think of my foods in terms of the type of carbohydrate molecule that composes them!). But they do summarize the specific carbohydrates that can be most likely to cause this form of GI discomfort.

FODMAP Diet:

All carbohydrates that are part of the FODMAP family are eliminated, which is a huge segment of the average person's dietary intake and includes various fruits, vegetables, and grains, as well as most forms of sugar and other sweeteners.

The reason that this acronym has become so popular is because of the diets built around it, often referred to as FODMAP diets in which all of these products are cut out completely. This can lead to a highly restrictive diet that is often not necessary, can be difficult to maintain, and can lead to nutrient deficiencies due to the extensive restriction. Unlike eliminating gluten from the diet of a person with Celiac disease, the FODMAP diet is not curative – it is simply meant to reduce symptoms.

There are breath tests available that can evaluate if you are sensitive to any specific carbohydrates in the FODMAP family, such as fructose. By having these breath tests conducted, you could identify whether you are truly sensitive to any FODMAP components and focus on removing only those from your diet. This would allow you to narrow down your sensitivities so that your dietary restrictions will be easier to maintain and less likely to impact your nutritional status.

If these breath tests do not identify any specific culprits, the FODMAP diet can be trialed. A permanent, strict FODMAP diet is rarely recommended because it is often not needed and can be so detrimental to long-term health. This dietary change can be tested for as little as a couple of weeks - if no change occurs in this time frame, then the diet does not work for you. If the diet does improve your symptoms, specific sugars can then be added back one at a time in order to identify the FODMAP component(s) that is the source of your symptoms.

Permanent use of a complete FODMAP diet is rarely recommended due to the difficulty in maintaining such a diet and the possibility for nutritional deficiencies. The actual problem carbohydrate(s) should be identified and should be the only ones permanently restricted from the diet.

NONCELIAC GLUTEN SENSITIVITY (NCGS)

We already discussed Celiac disease, a condition in which the body attacks itself due to an inappropriate reaction to gluten. The only treatment is the permanent and total elimination of gluten from the diet to halt the severe intestinal damage and the weight loss and nutrient deficiencies it can cause.

NCGS, on the other hand, describes the apparent existence of a sensitivity to gluten that does not result in actual intestinal damage. This very new concept has only recently emerged and is still poorly understood, although significant research is currently being conducted to improve our understanding.

We know so little about this condition that it is not even fully accepted as a true disorder within the medical community. There is also no test available to confirm whether it is present. The condition is actually defined as simply "an improvement in symptoms when gluten is removed from the diet and a recurrence of symptoms when it is added back in". The symptoms that have been attributed may be mild or severe and cover a large range, including bloating, gas, diarrhea, constipation, pain, nausea, fatigue, and mental fogginess.

One of the reasons that NCGS continues to be such a blurry concept is due to the number of people that have chosen to remove gluten from their diets without being tested for any other conditions. In fact, a gluten-free diet could be much more extreme than what is truly needed to improve a person's symptoms. It may also mask the actual cause of the problem. Many people that have improved on a gluten-free diet and then had proper testing completed were found to have a wide range of conditions, including fructose intolerance, SIBO, or microscopic colitis. Some of these conditions should be treated with medications or surgery and not recognizing their presence can lead to complications down the road.

Microscopic colitis is actually a further subdivision of IBD in which the inflammation of the colon causes persistent, watery diarrhea. This damage is treated with medications.

Again, I will reiterate that you should be tested for Celiac prior to removing gluten from your diet so that you can receive an accurate test result. Similarly, you should be tested for any of the conditions that we have already discussed (from IBS to carbohydrate sensitivity) before commencing a gluten-free diet. Proper testing for conditions that can be accurately diagnosed and treated is very important prior to implementing such a significant self-directed diet change. This approach will ensure that you are assessing all of your options and guaranteeing your best health.

A gluten-free diet may actually be a Band-Aid for a problem that requires medical treatment. If you think that something is wrong, insist that your doctor evaluate what it could be or refer you to someone that can.

Outside of possibly masking a more severe condition, a gluten-free diet carries concerns similar to those with the full FODMAP diet. Excessive restrictions are prone to result in nutritional deficiencies, a well-documented issue with gluten-free diets. Another concern that is present with these diets is that many commercially available gluten-free products are actually higher in sugar and fat than their traditional counterparts. This can make the diet even more difficult to follow if also trying to maintain a healthy and active lifestyle. Just as with the FODMAP diet, the gluten-free diet can be trialed for two weeks, at which point if it is not providing benefit, it should be considered ineffective.

ADDITIONAL GI CONCERNS: IN SUMMARY

It is possible that an additional GI disorder, such as IBS, Celiac, SIBO, or carbohydrate sensitivity, may be present for some people with gastroparesis. If the symptoms for these conditions mirror your own, then you should speak with your doctor about the possibility of obtaining the appropriate tests. In fact, if your doctor responds by telling you that you can try to modify your lifestyle based on symptoms and not on a diagnosis, he is doing you a disservice. If there is a possibility that you have any of these conditions, you have a right to insist on appropriate testing and diagnosis.

Defining exactly what is going on in our GI tracts is crucial to understanding the best way to treat and/or manage our symptoms. A proper diagnosis can provide a clearly marked path for diet modifications or medical treatments. Without this, any interventions may be misguided, which could be inconvenient at best and dangerous at worst.

I'd like to quickly circle back to the considerations we must also make for gastroparesis. Many of us would be doing ourselves a disservice to implement a highly restrictive diet on top of what, by nature, is an already limited diet. This could require us to remove highly nutritive foods that are actually well-tolerated. It may also require the elimination of a trusted 'comfort food', possibly leading to additional stress or anxiety during difficult times and situations.

To ensure that you are receiving the best care, you will have to be a diligent self-advocate that asks the right questions and makes the right changes

Concerns with restrictive diets:
1. Nutrient deficiencies
2. Difficulty to maintain
3. Increased sugar/fat intake
4. Cost

For those with gastroparesis, an additional risk involves eliminating go-to foods that are well tolerated with your delayed emptying and nausea. Any dietary restriction has the potential to cause stress and anxiety, which can compound with each additional restriction.

at the right times. Below is a general roadmap to follow regarding everything that we have covered with restrictive diets and GI conditions.

A roadmap within a roadmap!

But it's always the same idea: Think critically, evaluate your options, and move step-by-step, monitoring your progress closely.

1. **Do you believe that your symptoms might mirror any of those in the conditions discussed?**
   a. **No**: You can direct your focus on the management of gastroparesis and not deal with the distractions of these other considerations
   b. **Yes**: You should seek out a discussion with your doctor that specifically pinpoints the conditions that you are concerned for and why

2. **Does your doctor agree that it is possible that you have any of these other conditions in addition to your gastroparesis?**
   a. **No**: Make sure that you understand why he does not believe these conditions are present and ask if there is anything else that you should be considering
   b. **Yes**: You have a right and a responsibility to yourself to request that the appropriate tests be completed to confirm or deny the presence of said conditions

3. **Particularly in the case of Celiac disease, but also as a general rule, you should demand the appropriate testing be completed PRIOR to commencing diet changes or treatments**

4. **Did you discover that you do have one of these additional conditions?**
   a. **Yes**: Become familiar with this condition through research and discussion with your physician to understand what it means
      - Identify and thoroughly review your treatment options, ensuring that you implement these options only one at a time and carefully monitor your response to each (see page 26)
   b. **No**: You do not have any conditions that are identified upon testing, which may mean you only need to focus on your gastroparesis

- It is possible that you have an intolerance that cannot be directly tested, such as a member of the FODMAP family or a component of wheat. Dietary trials may be warranted to confirm or deny this.

5. **If the treatment for your diagnosed condition or possible sensitivity requires a change in diet**

   a. Request a referral to a registered dietician to ensure that your diet changes are well advised. A dietician will help you to avoid over-restriction, additional cost, or unwanted side effects such as nutritional deficiencies or increased sugar/fat intake

   b. Limit diet changes to no longer than a month. If it is going to work, it will work in that time frame. If no difference is noted, the change should be abandoned.

   c. For highly restrictive diets that do result in symptom improvement, insist upon paring down the diet one ingredient at a time so that you identify the least restrictive diet that works for you (i.e. add back one form of carbohydrate every 2 weeks)

ROADMAP SUMMARY

1. Identify a concern
2. Speak with your doctor
3. Get tested and diagnosed
4. Identify appropriate treatments as a result of a positive test and implement under guidance (physician or dietician, depending)
5. Identify possible options for issues that do not show up on tests, always focusing on the most likely and evidence-based causes and the healthiest and least-stressful management plan
6. Be responsible about the changes – implement one at a time and monitor your response closely

If an intervention doesn't lead to a positive change, abandon it!

THE LURE OF DIETARY EXPLANATIONS

You will find yourself constantly bombarded by a variety of special, restrictive diets. Many popular diets focus on the benefits of going 'back to our roots' or on eliminating one evil food group. These diets promise a fix for a whole variety of ailments, which is always an enticing proposition. Some may have a scientific basis and some may actually be helpful to a small number of people (such as those with fructose intolerance or Celiac disease), but many more will simply be ideas that stand to make a lot of money for a few and may be harmful for many. Protect yourself from dangerous claims and the frustration of implementing difficult changes with no payoff – utilize your knowledge for identifying appropriate resources and evaluating the information you find (see page 15). Always ask

"Does it sound too good to be true?" and "Does it make sense for me?".

Here are a couple of great quotes that can help to remind us to think sensibly before jumping in:

Going back to our roots actually means something different from every perspective!

Our bodies have adapted over time to different circumstances, including to cooking and to modern agriculture, and this process is always ongoing. There is no pristine virtue in what our ancestors ate in Paleolithic times, and in any case our bodies have already undergone significant changes since that time. Life, especially human life, is never perfectly matched to one kind of eating. It is always evolving as the food sources change.

- DIMITRA PAPAGIANNI, PhD (Paleontologist)

Tomatoes, peppers, squash, potatoes, avocados, pecans, cashews, and blueberries are all New World crops, and have only been on the dinner table of African and Eurasian populations for probably 10 generations of their evolutionary history. Europeans have been eating grain for the last 10,000 years; we've been eating sweet potatoes for less than 500. Yet the human body has seemingly adapted perfectly well to yams, let alone pineapple and sunflower seeds.

- KARL FENST (Bioarchaelogist)

CONCLUSION

This section was meant to improve your understanding for the many factors that can play a role in causing or worsening symptoms. Each of these factors has its associated treatments and interventions. Gastroparesis adds another layer of consideration with any such interventions and making questionable or difficult changes should not be taken lightly. Make sure that you always insist on the appropriate care from your medical team and the treatment that will be the most manageable and beneficial for you.

Personal Experience Part 6

Although I was still weakened, I was maintaining a better quality of life and felt suddenly empowered by the impact that I was able to have on my own condition. I was also beginning to feel more confident in my knowledge of health, diseases, and treatments through my education. And I suddenly realized – it had been 6 years since I got sick. This was past the allotted time that the previous doctor had stated was preventing my candidacy for the neurostimulator. My accomplishments in improving my own health allowed me to rebuild my motivation to tackle the healthcare system again.

When I had previously pushed to see various doctors and obtain different treatments, I was more interested in having my gastroparesis "fixed". However, after a discouraging and fruitless journey that eventually ended with introspection, I was now convinced that the neurostimulator was simply an additional instrument in my efforts to regain an acceptable quality of life. And I finally understood that even if the neurostimulator was beneficial to me, I would never be "fixed". I would have to continue to employ my lifestyle changes and be an active participant in taking care of myself, or it would fail to make a true difference.

So I set out on my mission to get a neurostimulator. At first I went back to that physician in San Francisco. Well, it turned out that in the 3 years since I had seen him last, he had moved on from the neurostimulator and was now researching a few different medications. He said that he was more interested in enrolling me in his medication studies and didn't want to implant the neurostimulator. The repeat interaction with this doctor and the continued hopelessness that he presented for me hit me very hard – I initially became quite discouraged and depressed by his response.

But I quickly bounced back and began looking at my other options. I found another doctor that was actually closer to home that had recently started implanting neurostimulators. And in so doing found the doctor that, to this day, is still the best doctor that I have ever had the honor of seeing. He was incredibly compassionate. He took the time to understand me, my symptoms, my concerns, and my history. He listened to the changes that I had made and my reasons for wanting the stimulator. He ordered a few tests so that he could get a current evaluation of my condition, and he recommended some additional strategies that I had not tried, such as liquid protein.

When my test results came back, they showed that I still had severely delayed emptying that had not improved since my previous tests 3 and 4 years before. He agreed that considering the stable and severe nature of my delay and my persistent symptoms, the neurostimulator was my best option and brought his surgeon on board to review my chart and agree to the placement. I was thrilled that I had finally discovered such a compassionate doctor with whom I felt that I had established a real relationship. I was even more thrilled when I found out that they were going to try to do something to help! And then the bad news came – my insurance wouldn't approve the stimulator.

I set about writing letters back and forth to my insurance company, explaining my symptoms and my needs and pleading with them to approve the placement. I even used some of what I was learning in pharmacy school to make the case that they would save money in the future by preventing hospital and emergency room visits, but to no avail. I was denied over and over again. But this time, instead of feeling depressed, it made me angry. I was beginning to develop a real passion regarding the way that our healthcare system was run and how many times I had been denied the treatment or attention that I needed to improve my quality of life.

So I changed insurance companies. I spoke with my doctor to find out which plans had approved it in the past and was incredibly lucky to discover that I had access to one of those plans during open enrollment. The cost of the insurance was higher, but in the end that would be a small price to pay for coverage. And suddenly the claim flew through with no issue – I was approved and the surgery was scheduled!

I allowed myself to be happy and excited for a few days before beginning to plan for the surgery and the recovery. This was a huge step in the right direction. There was always a chance that the neurostimulator wouldn't work for me, but I knew that I had done everything else that I could at this point and had to take that risk in hopes of further improving my quality of life. I was only 22 and quite concerned about what my future would hold in the long term if I continued to be as sick as I had been. I had long ago mentally committed myself to this process, and I knew that the most challenging part of that process was still awaiting me – recovering after the surgery.

Alternative Therapies, Part One 8

"Nature has no bias and can be seen at work as clearly, and as inexorably, in the spread of an epidemic as in the birth of a healthy baby."

MEDICAL MONITOR

We have one more large, foundational topic to discuss in order to thoroughly round out the information provided in the first section of this book. That topic, as you can see from the chapter title, is Alternative Therapies. By this I am referring to dietary supplements, nutrient supplementation, diet enhancing products, herbal products, herbal treatments, natural alternatives, Eastern medicines, and any and all products and therapies that fall under the general heading of "Alternative or Complementary Treatments".

WHAT ARE ALTERNATIVE THERAPIES?

The first thing that we need to do is define our topic. I just listed a bunch of examples of Alternative Therapies, but in a more general sense, the name itself implies where these options fall within the typical world of treatments and therapies – "other". These are the alternative options because they are not typically accepted, recommended, or encouraged by the traditional medical system.

But this is not because doctors and the medical system have something to lose by turning to these treatment options, or because there is some type of vendetta held between practitioner types. It is simply this:

The evidence and information necessary to show that these treatments work and are safe for people to use consistently is lacking.

Hippocrates, the father of modern Western medicine, once wrote, "As to diseases, make a habit of two things – to help, or at least to do no harm." In this case, recommending alternative therapies would not allow physicians to follow this basic tenet of medicine, as they cannot be sure that these therapies are in the best interest of their patients and will do them no harm.

Alternative therapies are those therapies that are not considered 'proven' to be safe and effective for use.

If an alternative therapy is adequately studied and shown to work, it is often adopted by the medical system.

Gastroparesis is a condition that is not curable and in many ways is not fully treatable by the medical system. We fall into that category of patients that get bounced around from doctor to test to doctor and often walk away with less to wrap our hopes around than we need. It is only natural and logical for us to seek out alternative options that might provide some form of hope or relief. After all, I keep saying that we are ultimately responsible for our own health, right?

I am not saying that it's Western medicine or nothing! In fact, we will discuss these topics in much more detail in the following pages. I will dig into the information that is available for many of these alternative therapies. I will also discuss the ways that you can protect yourself by ensuring that some of these alternatives are safe for you to use. As with every other section of this book, my goal here is to make sure that you are a fully informed patient and consumer, able to evaluate the information in a way that allows you to both improve and protect your own health.

I hope that each person can come into this conversation with an open mind and consider all of the information, just as I did. So let's dive in!

"NON-ALTERNATIVE THERAPY" OVERSIGHT

The best way to understand why something is considered an alternative therapy is to first understand what makes something a non-alternative, or traditional, therapy. While I am going to speak to the structure that is currently established in the United States, the concepts and general process that we will review hold true for most countries around the world.

MEDICATIONS

Medications can only be marketed in the United States if they have obtained approval from the Food and Drug Administration (FDA). This includes over-the-counter medications, as well as those that are obtained via a prescription, or behind the counter. The process to obtain FDA approval is fairly rigorous, and requires the investment of significant time and money from the companies that sell these medications to consumers. Let's take a quick stroll through that process:

Over-the-Counter (OTC): Available on the drugstore shelf

Prescription (Rx Only): Only available from behind the counter, with a prescription

Drug discovery: This is the very beginning of the process, when scientists evaluate different molecules in a lab to see if they have a desired impact on human cells. In recent years, this process has become more streamlined through newly available tests and our growing understanding of the human genome.

Hundreds of molecules can be screened before a single promising molecule is identified

Animal testing: Once a molecule is considered promising, it will typically be tested on certain types of animals. The type of animal will vary depending on what disease or symptom is being treated – scientists will attempt to utilize the animal that mimics that condition in humans.

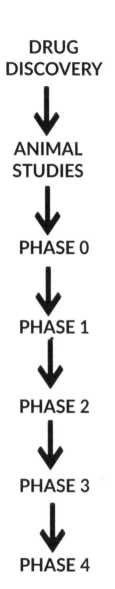

DRUG DISCOVERY

↓

ANIMAL STUDIES

↓

PHASE 0

↓

PHASE 1

↓

PHASE 2

↓

PHASE 3

↓

PHASE 4

WHEN ALL IS SAID AND DONE, A MOLECULE THAT MADE IT THROUGH ANIMAL STUDIES HAS ONLY A 5-10% CHANCE OF BECOMING FDA APPROVED

This is the part of the process that sometimes leads to outrageous news articles like "Scientists have cured diabetes!". Reporters jump on information coming from a very early stage animal study and sensationalize it by representing it incorrectly. It is good to be wary of these stories because, as you will see, they are very unlikely to result in any actual treatments for humans.

Animal testing can take years to complete, and many previously promising molecules will be abandoned before reaching human studies

---

Phase 0 Studies: If a drug shows success in animal studies, the company that is studying the molecule can apply for approval from the FDA to begin testing in humans. Once approval is obtained, this short phase is entered and the molecule will be tested for the first time in a very small number of humans in an effort to evaluate how the body processes it.

Phase I Studies: Typically conducted in healthy people, these small studies have a primary goal of gaining a better understanding regarding what doses may be needed in humans, how long the drug stays in the body, and also where it goes in the body. These studies usually only include about 20–50 people.

TIME: 1–2 YEARS / COST: $10 MILLION

70% of molecules that made it to Phase I testing will successfully move on

---

Phase II Studies: These are typically the first studies to be conducted in people that have the condition that is being treated. A few selected doses will be tested in these studies in an effort to evaluate whether the medication actually leads to the desired effect. This is also the first time that side effects are observed and recorded in a standardized manner.

TIME: 2 YEARS / COST $20 MILLION

Only 33% of molecules successfully move past Phase II

Phase III Studies: These are the final phase of studies that are conducted prior to obtaining FDA approval. These trials are typically very large – thousands of patients – and attempt to confirm or deny that the molecule being studied does lead to the desired change. Remember our discussion about the Randomized Controlled Trial (RCT) being the gold standard? (see page 20) This is where a large number of those RCTs come from. Although it is never the primary goal of these studies, they are also required to rigorously evaluate side effects and potential negative outcomes that a molecule might cause.

TIME: 3-4 YEARS / COST: $45 MILLION

Only 25-30% of molecules that go in to Phase III will come out as a success

---

FDA Approval: At this point, if a drug shows true benefit that outweighs the possible harm after extensive testing, then the company can apply for FDA approval to make the drug available for use in the United States.

This is the goal of the FDA in their regulation of medications: Drugs that provide a true possibility of benefit that outweighs the possibility of harm.

TIME: 1-2 YEARS

Phase IV: This phase involves us – the point at which you and I might actually be taking this drug because it was prescribed by a doctor. All approved medications are extensively monitored by the FDA and constantly evaluated for new concerns that could not be identified in those earlier studies. This is yet another example of how medical practice improves and changes with experience (see page 23). As more people take a medication over a longer period of time, we have larger numbers that allow us to see things that might only occur rarely (1 in a million) or with prolonged use (over years instead of months). As soon as a new safety issue is identified, the FDA will send out alerts and attempt to find ways to reduce this risk.

A small percentage of approved drugs will end up not succeeding after all; we are all aware of drugs that have been pulled from the market because a serious, unexpected risk was found

---

If you are interested in a riveting story and the opportunity to learn more about what the FDA has done for our national health (it does get a pretty bad rap most of the time), I highly recommend Protecting America's Health: The FDA, Business, and 100 Years of Regulation by Phillip Hilts.

Once a medication has made it through this long and tedious process, it is still under tight regulation and scrutiny. One form of scrutiny is what I just referred to as Phase IV. Another form of scrutiny is the standard that the FDA holds for the manufacturing plants that make and distribute these medications. These standards are called Good Manufacturing Practices (GMP) and ensure that when you take a medication, you can be certain of the following:

- The drug you are holding is the drug listed on the bottle

- The dose of the drug is exactly the dose listed on the bottle

- The ingredients of the product are exactly what you were told they were

- There are no other drugs included in the product

- There are no contaminants (heavy metals, pesticides) in the product

- There are no infectious organisms (bacteria, fungus) in the product

By regulating our medications in the United States, the FDA has made every effort to guarantee us that any appropriately prescribed medication has been shown to have a benefit, that if there are possible negative effects involved, they are not greater than the possible benefit, and that we will not be put at risk by the way that the medication was manufactured.

NON-DRUG INTERVENTIONS

There are a number of different medical interventions that do not involve drugs. The ones with which we are most familiar are medical devices (i.e. a cardiac defibrillator), surgeries (i.e. hip replacement), and lifestyle modifications (i.e. calorie reduction for weight loss).

The regulation of medical devices in the United States is also conducted by the FDA. Although not identical to the rigorous process required for medications, devices must also prove to be beneficial and low risk. In addition, the FDA strictly regulates the manufacturing and quality assurance related to these devices in order to prevent unwanted adverse effects or malfunctions.

As you might imagine, other interventions like surgeries and lifestyle modifications do not really require approval by a regulating body. In fact, they can't even be studied in the same way that one specific medication or one specific device can be evaluated. However, they can still be studied, and there are endless such studies out there that have been conducted in an effort to evaluate the risks and benefits of these types of interventions.

When non-medication interventions become a standard part of medicine, this is because high quality studies have shown that they do lead to a benefit and do not have enough risk to offset that benefit. In fact, these same outcomes have typically been repeated in different studies, further validating that finding. When this happens, the findings are incorporated into standard practice and often included in medical guidelines. Guidelines exist in all medical specialties to help guide doctors through the treatments and interventions that have been shown to provide benefit with limited risk.

Being aware of the possible negative effects that can occur with the use of a medication is often taken for granted.

While we tend to look at that list of side effects and think "Wow, drugs are dangerous", we should try to shift our thinking to "Wow, I am lucky to have all of this information so that I can make an informed decision and be aware of possible issues."

The media is often to blame for this negative focus on adverse reactions. It is rare to see a headline like "Drug continues to work in millions of people!" attract the attention of a headline like "Drug might be causing liver failure!"

All of the discussion that we just had about medications and non-medication interventions represents something called evidence-based medicine. When physicians practice evidence-based medicine, it ensures that they are providing their patients with the highest likelihood for health and improvement, and the lowest likelihood for risks. Utilizing the results of studies or the guidelines that have been developed based on these studies, doctors can consider their patient's needs and situations and work in a step-by-step progression to reduce the risk of harm to their patients. As therapies fail, doctors can then move on to other options, each usually with slightly more risk or less chance of benefit. When riskier options are used, it is because the safer options have not worked and the risk is worthwhile to the patient in exchange for the possible benefit.

We just took a whirlwind tour through the basics of treatment regulation and the way that evidence is used to inform the practice of medicine in the United States. Many of you may already be drilling down that information mentally and seeing how it relates to some of your previous negative experiences. What we had before was an overview of the forest, and later on in the book we will give appropriate time and attention to the individual trees. But for better or worse, we have established that our government and medical community are pushing forward with the focus of providing the most benefits with the least risk.

ALTERNATIVE THERAPY OVERSIGHT

The path that the United States took to reach our current state of drug and intervention oversight was a difficult, long, and deadly one. As the Smithsonian pharmacy historian, Michael R. Harris, once stated, "The story of drug regulation is built on tombstones." And yet we have entered an era in which we take the state of our regulatory

The highest likelihood of benefit and the lowest likelihood of unwanted effects follows this progression:

Benefits >> Risks
Benefits > Risks
Benefits ≥ Risks
Benefits = Risks
Benefits ≤ Risks

This progression is done in conjunction with the patient, and only with their agreement that the risk is worth the possible reward.

I'll be the first to admit that we sometimes fail at this effort, particularly through the eyes of someone with a chronic disease. But that is not for lack of trying, and it is most definitely not what happens in the majority of cases.

Although we always hear about the failures and the bad experiences, we are constantly benefiting from all of the successes of modern medicine and the times that they got it right!

The experience of a person with a chronic condition can be particularly disheartening and foster disdain for the medical profession. I know – I've been there. But don't let this experience push you to leap blindly into uncharted territory with alternative therapies, where the risks might actually be higher with even more limited reward.

system for granted, expecting to be protected from the most egregious of harms and from the ill intentions of others whenever possible.

The logical conclusion to be drawn from everything that we just covered is that alternative therapies must fall under this same oversight. In fact, a recent Harris poll found that 68% of our population believes that the government requires herbal manufacturers to report side effects, and 58% believe that the FDA must approve herbal products before sale.

What if I told you that both of those statements are frighteningly far from the truth? Then you might ask something like, "Fine, so how are alternative therapies regulated?" And I would cringe and say, "The simple answer? They're not."

As we move forward in our discussion, we will see with increasing clarity that this is the point at which alternative therapies deviate from the traditional, non-alternative therapies that we just reviewed.

WILD AND WONDERFUL OR THE WILD WEST?

It took us a little while to walk through the steps involved in bringing a medication to the market. The good news here is that when we are talking about alternative therapies, the discussion will be much quicker – there is no process.

If any person wanted to sell an alternative therapy of their creation, they could do just that. They don't need to worry about conducting studies to see if it works, or to evaluate whether or not it's safe. In fact, they don't even have to show that what they're selling you is actually what they say they are selling. So instead of discussing the evaluation process as we did with medications, we are going to discuss why there is no evaluation process at all for alternative therapies and what that means for us.

There are actually a number of somewhat frightening videos online that demonstrate how incredibly easy it is to make and market a supplement.

Back in 1994, something called the Dietary Supplement Health and Education Act (DSHEA) was passed into law. This Act was the result of extensive lobbying on the part of the dietary supplement and herbals market. It gained widespread public acceptance because it was sold to our nation as the only way to keep the government from banning our vitamins. When I talk about the implications of DSHEA, I am referring to the products that fall into its definition:

A dietary supplement is a product intended for ingestion that contains a "dietary ingredient" intended to add further nutritional value to (supplement) the diet. Dietary supplements may be found in many forms such as tablets, capsules, softgels, gelcaps, liquids, or powders. A "dietary ingredient" may be one, or any combination, of the following substances:

- *A vitamin*
- *A mineral*
- *An herb or other botanical*
- *An amino acid*
- *A dietary substance for use by people to supplement the diet by increasing the total dietary intake*
- *A concentrate, metabolite, constituent, or extract*

As you can see, a dietary supplement in this case includes a wide array of products that could loosely fall within this category. But one aspect of this definition is clear – these are all products that can be taken by mouth. As such, they are commonly confused with medications and assumed to fall under the same type of regulatory control. Another point of confusion for many people is the realization that vitamins fall under this category. The multivitamins that we grew up taking on a daily basis, the Vitamin D and calcium that many of us take now, and even the B Vitamins that the doctor has recommended to balance out our restricted diets – these are all considered dietary supplements.

The essence of DSHEA was to create a separate category for these products that could not be regulated by the FDA. In other words, it took away the accountability that comes with regulation by a third party. For all intents and purposes, it placed the people that are making and selling these products in charge of ensuring the product's safety, quality, and efficacy. This means that none of the safeguards that we discussed earlier that ensure that our medications are safe and effective are in place for alternative therapies. In fact, the FDA can only intervene after a serious health event has occurred. In other words, many people must be harmed before our government can jump in to protect the health of our country.

This is similar to leaving a child in charge of policing their own media consumption and expecting it to be done appropriately.

While it would be nice to believe that the people producing natural and alternative therapies have the best of intentions, history has shown otherwise. Below is a brief overview of the major events that have occurred since the passage of DSHEA. You will note that as the medical community became more aware that risks existed with these products, they began to apply a higher level of scrutiny, resulting in a snowballing of concerns.

And you know what they say about good intentions...

1994: Various ginseng products were tested and found to contain no ginseng at all, far less than stated, or far more than stated

This list includes only a sampling of issues from each year. There are many, many more where these came from.

1997: An herbal product claiming to contain kava, a plant from the western Pacific, was found to not contain any trace of this ingredient

1998: Upon testing 16 products claiming to contain a supplement called DHEA (dehydroepiandrosterone; used to boost sex drive and build muscle), only 7 actually contained the quantity stated and 3 contained no DHEA at all

1998: Various tested dietary supplements were found to be contaminated with digitalis, a potentially fatal molecule used in the prescription drug, digoxin

2004: After 8 years of fighting, the FDA was finally allowed to ban the inclusion of ephedra from any product sold in the United States

- By the time that the FDA was able to succeed with the ban, there were over 17,000 official reports of severe toxicity from ephedra, which included 155 known deaths

- Ephedra was included in products marketed for weight loss and enhanced performance

- Its use was clearly associated with increased blood pressure, heart attack, stroke, seizure, and sudden death

- Ephedra-containing products can still be purchased online

2007: The FDA was permitted to begin auditing a small number of supplement manufacturers and found that "some didn't use recipes for their products, some substituted ingredients on a whim, and some facilities were contaminated with rodent feces and urine"

2009: The FDA received over 130 reports that a Zicam intranasal cold remedy had caused a complete loss of smell with use, leading them to warn the company that the product must be pulled from the shelves

- The company that made Zicam had already received an additional 800 complaints but had taken no action

- The loss of smell was permanent in a large percentage of the people affected

2010: An independent study conducted by the Government Accountability Office (GAO) found that 16 of 40 tested supplements contained pesticide residues exceeding the legal limits

2013: Upon testing 44 herbal products, 59% were found to contain plants that were not on the label, 33% contained contaminants and fillers that were not on the label, and only 2 out of 12 companies produced products that were true to the label, uncontaminated, and undiluted

2013: When testing 15 different bottles of Vitamin D (cholecalciferol) it was found that they contained anywhere from 52-135% of the amount stated on the label

2013: A supplement product called OxyElite Pro was found to contain a new, untested dietary ingredient named aegeline that was associated with at least 93 cases of non-viral hepatitis, 47 hospitalizations, 3 liver transplants, and 1 death

2013: A B-vitamin complex supplement was found to be contaminated with anabolic steroids, which caused at least 29 reported toxicities, including hair loss, muscle cramping, and liver injury

2015: A study indicated that dietary supplements are responsible for >20,000 emergency room visits annually, for symptoms such as nausea and vomiting, allergic reactions, and heart trouble

2015: The New York Attorney General called for 13 companies to remove their products from shelves in the state of New York after testing showed that they did not contain the ingredients on the label

2016: A study showed that 1 in 5 cases of liver failure is now caused by herbal and dietary supplements, up from 1 in 10 cases ten years ago

You will notice in the above timeline that 2013 might have signaled somewhat of a death knell for the dietary supplement industry. In that year alone, there were 42 cases of product quality issues that resulted in an FDA-mandated recall, usually due to supplements containing a prescription drug that was not listed on the label (this is in addition to what is shown in the timeline above). In the same year, the institution that I worked for attempted to evaluate the quality of the supplements that

Don't worry, I won't ignore the other side of this: Prescription drugs were responsible for far more ER visits than that.

The major difference is that doctors are able to quickly identify what caused a drug-related problem and also know how to quickly address it.

Visits related to supplements are sometimes left as unreported mysteries because products might have been contaminated or a patient might not have even thought to tell the doctor that they were taking a supplement at all. (Always let a doctor, pharmacist, or nurse know what supplements you are taking in addition to any prescribed medication!)

And finally, while prescription drugs are taken for a legitimate medical need, supplement use is often optional. This makes the risk-benefit breakdown difficult to justify when it lands a person in the hospital.

we were providing to our hospitalized patients, only to discover that these supplements contained anywhere from 70-250% of the amount of the ingredient listed on the label. An FDA inspector was quoted as saying that at least 70% of the manufacturers surveyed in the past 5 years "...have run afoul of the US FDA's manufacturing regulations".

Ok, so let's take a quick step back. I mentioned that dietary supplements are considered to be in a class of their own, and this class is not subject to FDA oversight. The only time that the FDA can step in is after the occurrence of a negative event. While the manufacturers of dietary supplements claim to have only the best of intentions in improving the health of the people that use their products, this does not appear true on close examination.

In the timeline above, we highlighted only the largest news stories that implicated dietary supplements. Many smaller stories are not included here, and many stories were never recognized or reported at all. It is also very important to note that when one side effect to a product is reported, it is appropriate to assume that there are at least 10-100 *more* unreported events. All of that being said, the information that we've looked at is very concerning. And although 2013 should likely have signaled a change for the industry, the market for supplements has only continued to grow. Supplements, natural therapies, and herbal products continue to be portrayed in a positive light and sought out as a desirable alternative to the drugs of Western medicine.

I am not trying to say that all supplements are evil and only FDA-approved drugs are good. In fact, I will openly admit that many FDA-approved drugs can be dangerous. The difference is that we know when those drugs are dangerous because we have studied those dangers. Dietary supplements, on the other hand, are unknowns. Due to the current lack of regulation and oversight, the greatest concern with these therapies is the

The dangers of the unknown:

Unknown toxicity
Unknown benefit
Unknown ingredients

unknown – unknown toxicity, unknown benefit, and unknown ingredients.

ALL HOPE IS NOT LOST

It is important to recognize that whether we like it or not, many of the herbal and supplemental products on the market (those touted as 'all natural') are not typically what they claim to be.

First of all, they do not necessarily even contain the ingredient that is stated on the label. There might be a large, small, or nonexistent amount of said ingredient in any given product.

Secondly, an unexpected ingredient might also be in the product. This could be another supplement or herbal ingredient, or it could even be a prescription drug. For those with food allergies, it may be an allergen that you need to avoid.

Thirdly, the product might contain contaminants in the form of pesticides, chemicals, and heavy metals. Various studies have shown that many supplements contain unacceptable levels of these unwanted ingredients.

But I promise – not all hope is lost! While limited, there is a way to ensure that the product that you are buying does not carry one or all of the three concerns listed above. This is through third-party certification.

I had mentioned that the FDA has specific standards that drug manufacturers must follow to ensure that the medications you are taking are exactly what you expect them to be and are not contaminated (see page 110). Third-party certification acts as this missing step for the supplement industry. Unfortunately, this certification is entirely voluntary. This fact is a double-edged sword – while only a small number of products will hold third-party certification, the certification acts as a clear badge of integrity for the product and the company seeking it out.

I want to reiterate here that I have no disclosures. I have never worked for or received payments from any of the certifiers or companies listed in this book.

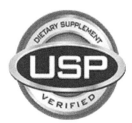

The **United States Pharmacopeia (USP)** is the highest badge available for a dietary supplement product. Their badge is called USP-Verified and will be clearly affixed to any tested products. USP holds any verified products to a standard matching what would be expected of a prescription drug being monitored by the FDA. In fact, USP even conducts random off-the-shelf testing of bottles to ensure that the company is maintaining the quality of products between audits. I personally find that particular fact to be very reassuring. If a product holds USP Verification, then you know it is not contaminated with unwanted ingredients and that it contains the ingredient that is on the label, in the quantity that is listed on the label.

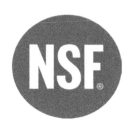

The **National Science Foundation (NSF)** also maintains a third-party certification program for supplements. The major difference here is that NSF Certification is done for the manufacturer, not for individual products. This means that you might find a stamp of approval on the company website, but not necessarily on the bottle that you find on the shelf. It is a highly stringent certification and holds the same value as USP Verification, but it is more difficult to identify. NSF does conduct certification for some individual products, but it is limited to exercise-enhancing supplements, a market that is less likely to impact those of us with gastroparesis.

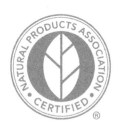

The **Natural Products Association (NPA)** also conducts a voluntary third-party certification for interested manufacturers. However, this certification does not hold the same standard as would be expected through USP and NSF. NPA conducts audits only once every two years and does not perform any random audits off-the-shelf. Additionally, NPA Certification is only conducted for manufacturers, not for specific products. So again, you might find a stamp of approval on the company website, but not on the bottle on the shelf.

Here we have three solid options for ensuring that any supplements or herbal products that you purchase will not be harmful to you because of the way that they were manufactured. We have already established that this is a real concern, so implementing this additional layer of care when purchasing a product is something that I strongly advocate to all hospitals and consumers. Of the options above, USP is the clear winner for both its high standards and easily identified labeling. NSF is a close second place, simply because it is not as easy to identify. NPA does not represent the same quality as the previous two, but it does represent a higher standard than those products that hold no certification whatsoever.

Many of you might be actively checking the supplements that you currently own, or Googling the ones that you would like to buy. Many of you might soon discover that it is not as easy as one might like to identify products that hold these certifications. However, I do encourage you to take the extra time to find a product that has been verified by a third party in order to protect your health and safety. While the recent news and production surrounding the dietary supplement industry has not impacted its sales, more and more companies have begun to participate in certification programs to send a message to consumers that their products are different. As this trend continues, it will not only improve the quality of the products on the market, but also make it easier for the informed shopper to find products that are safe to use.

Why am I spending so much time talking about this? Because as of 4 years ago, I wasn't aware of any of it and only encountered it accidentally through my job. In fact, most pharmacists and physicians do not even know the extent of the concerns, and word is slow to spread.

Recent polls indicate that 60% of people in the United States believe that supplements are wholly regulated by the FDA – in quality, safety, and efficacy. It appears it is becoming ever more dangerous for this misunderstanding to continue.

You may eventually come across an ingredient that you want to try that is not made by a single company that holds a third party certification. It may be tempting in this case to just go ahead and buy it anyways. But this dilemma actually leads us into the next part of our discussion on alternative therapies regarding their safety and efficacy. So hold that thought and let's dive into this topic further.

Alternative Therapies, Part Two 9

"*Exaggerated claims for the efficacy of a medicament are very seldom the consequence of any intention to deceive; they are usually the outcome of a kindly conspiracy in which everybody has the very best intentions. The patient wants to get well, his physician wants to have made him better, and the pharmaceutical company would have liked to have put it into the physician's power to have made him so. The controlled clinical trial is an attempt to avoid being taken in by this conspiracy of good will.*"

SIR PETER MEDAWAR

Now that we know how to avoid the pitfalls of a poorly made dietary supplement, we can expand our discussion to the potential for benefits and risks with alternative therapies as a whole. We have hardly had a chance thus far to put our knowledge about Levels of Evidence and evidence quality into action (see page 20). That is about to change!

We already know that FDA drug regulation requires the completion of high quality research and studies to show that a medication does have a real benefit. These same studies also thoroughly evaluate the risks and side effects associated with that drug, which is factored into its overall value. The FDA is tasked with making a final determination regarding the benefit-risk ratio for that drug and ensuring that the public is aware of any safety concerns that might occur alongside the desired benefit.

Let's expand on our knowledge so that we can conduct our best version of this process for the alternative therapies that are not evaluated by the FDA.

CONDUCTING THE APPROPRIATE STUDIES

We can take this opportunity to develop a deeper understanding of how our gold standard studies are conducted and the ways that they are structured to improve their validity. It's time to talk about the placebo (see page 69).

Placebo is Latin for "I will please"

A placebo can come in various forms and its effect can manifest in many, sometimes surprising, ways. I hold true to my previous statement that the placebo effect is a fascinating topic that deserves attention in a book of its own. I will limit my discussion here to what we need to consider about the placebo effect for our own health and well-being and how the medical profession attempts to incorporate it into the practice of evidence-based medicine.

The first important point to recognize is that any treatment, proven or not, can elicit a placebo effect. In fact, the simple act of a doctor prescribing a medication and implying that it will help – possibly providing some eye contact and verbal reassurance at the same time – has been shown to positively impact the effect that medication has on the person taking it. Our brains are powerful things! The second important point to recognize dovetails off of this one. If just the act of giving someone a medication can lead to some type of improvement, then how can you possibly tell if the medication or treatment is actually working or if it's just the placebo effect in action?

Some less important, but fun placebo points?

- An injection has a bigger placebo effect than a pill
- A large pill has a bigger effect than a small pill
- Yellow pills seem to work better than others in the treatment of depression
- Fancy branding on a package has a larger effect than plain, boring packaging

We have discussed the exceptional value of the randomized controlled trial and the fact that it is considered the gold standard. One of the ways that the RCT attains such a high level of evidence deals specifically with how it combats the placebo effect. A randomized controlled trial is exactly what the name states – randomized and controlled. The study is split into different arms that utilize different interventions, including the treatment of interest (we'll refer to it in this case as Intervention Y) and, most commonly, a placebo. The arm of

Randomized: Randomly places participants into different arms of the study

Controlled: Includes a 'control' arm that does not use the Intervention that is being studied. This allows us to evaluate if it is the actual Intervention making a difference or simply a placebo-type effect

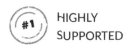 HIGHLY SUPPORTED

the study that is not receiving Intervention Y is referred to as the 'control'. The people that enter the study are then randomized – randomly placed – into either the treatment arm or the control arm.

This all sounds fine and many of you are probably already familiar with these concepts. So we are comparing an intervention to a placebo and that makes sense. This way we know if people got better simply because they received any type of treatment at all, regardless of whether it was Intervention Y. But how would you be able to see that effect unless the person in the study didn't actually know that they were taking a placebo instead of Intervention Y? The technique that is used to combat this confounding issue is called 'blinding'. The people in a study are not aware of which treatment they are receiving. So if the only benefit that is seen is from the placebo effect, then technically the people in both arms of the study should have the same level of response.

Blinding: The participant does not know if they are receiving the intervention or a placebo. The placebo is made to appear identical in every way to the actual intervention.

But it doesn't stop there. The most well-designed studies implement something termed 'double-blinding'. This goes one step further in that the doctor is also blinded regarding whether the patient is receiving Intervention Y or the placebo. Why? Because doctors are not immune to the placebo effect – in fact, no one is. Doctors could act differently around the people that they know are receiving Intervention Y, or they could infer certain expectations to people that they know are receiving the placebo. They could be more encouraging to those that are receiving Intervention Y, or they could even go so far as to exaggerate study results that are subjective. Regardless of whether it is the result of good intentions, it must still be addressed in order to prevent incorrect conclusions.

Double-blinding: Neither the participant nor the doctor knows if the participant is receiving the intervention or the placebo.

So why bring this up now? Because the placebo effect is particularly important to consider when evaluating alternative therapies. Many of the original studies that were conducted on alternative therapies did not consider the impact of the placebo effect at all. In fact, they even sometimes compared a group of patients receiving an intervention to a group of patients left on a waiting list. The science used to evaluate alternative therapies has gotten much better in the past couple of decades, but it is important to be aware that those types of studies are out there, and are often touted by people that want to convince others of the benefit of a certain intervention.

We'll keep an eye out for these as we discuss specific therapies, just as you will as you move forward to evaluating your options on your own.

Another important consideration is that it is sometimes difficult to identify an appropriate placebo for certain forms of alternative therapy. For instance, it might be hard to imagine a placebo option for the needle insertion necessary for acupuncture. It is also difficult to dream up a way to appropriately evaluate the power of healing touch or Reiki. But have no fear – someone got there before us!

Many governments have actually been directing grant funding specifically towards the study of alternative therapies for some time now. The United States has an entire branch of our National Institutes of Health (NIH) dedicated to this research, called the National Center for Complementary and Integrative Health (NCCIH) . Thanks to these funding efforts and focused attention on evaluating alternative therapies, we have strong, placebo-controlled studies allowing us to discern whether or not many alternative therapies are effective.

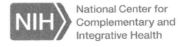

National Center for Complementary and Integrative Health

POOLED STUDIES

There is one final type of evidence evaluation that bears mentioning before we jump into looking at different forms of alternative therapies. I probably sound like a broken record at this point from all of the times that I have said "the more numbers, the better", or "the more studies that show the same result, the more valid the finding". But mine is not the only broken record and scientists have developed a way to evaluate these growing numbers and findings clearly – systematic reviews and meta-analyses.

Systematic reviews pull together all available studies on a certain topic and consider their level of evidence (high quality or not). They then piece together the findings of these studies to come to a final conclusion on the effect of a certain intervention. A meta-analysis also pulls together all studies on a certain topic. But the statistician conducting this meta-analysis will go one step further – they will pool all of the data from these studies together and then run the numbers again. In short, these two types of reviews allow us to take a high-resolution snapshot of the information that currently exists on a topic and obtain a clear picture for the level of evidence that is pointing in one direction or the other.

BENEFITS AND RISKS: NATURAL/HERBAL/ DIETARY SUPPLEMENTS

We've already hit the ground running with these products, so why not tackle them first as we move from product quality to benefits and risks. We know that the FDA doesn't regulate these products and doesn't evaluate whether or not they are safe or effective. So the burden falls on us as consumers to conduct this evaluation, an evaluation that will be much easier for some products than others.

Unfortunately, I would be doing everyone a disservice if I made an effort to exhaustively list the benefits and risks of the various natural remedies that are available on the market. This is partly because it would be an impossible task for me to relay information on all pertinent products within the confines of this book. It is also partly because that information changes with time. It could be that very few studies for a certain product will exist at the time that this book goes to print, but five years later there will be adequate evidence to draw a conclusion regarding benefits and risks.

Compendiums are available that do a fantastic job of compiling, evaluating, and summarizing the current evidence base for a plethora of natural supplements and herbal products. In fact, the Natural Standard Herb and Supplement Guide includes information on more than 400 ingredients. This is not limited to just the studies that have been conducted – it includes reports of toxicities and concerns specific to each product's purity and dose. Warnings and precautions for certain age groups and specific medical conditions, including pregnancy, are also provided. It may be possible to find this compendium at a local library to reduce the cost.

For instance, did you know that the stem of the kava flower is the most common cause for liver toxicity? Products that are purified to contain only the petal are much less likely to carry this risk.

Alternatively, this compendium is available in a continuously updated, fully searchable, online format as well. It is called the Natural Medicine Comprehensive Database and includes all of the information found in the Natural Standard, except with the additional inclusion of the most recently available risk and benefit information. This website can be accessed for a minimal fee that can be easily justified when compared to the cost of the average supplement product. For further cost savings, consider activating and deactivating the subscription to accommodate your needs as a consumer and patient.

As of 2017, this fee was $15/ month with only a monthly commitment required.

In the pages of these resources, you will find products which do have adequate information available to distinguish between those that are helpful and those that are harmful (and be forewarned – you will find that many have been deemed harmful). But there are also products that will have an unknown designation, or worse yet, will not be found within those resources at all. It is those supplements that have not undergone the necessary testing and have not been adequately studied for which the risks are greatest. In the time between having no knowledge and having adequate knowledge regarding risks and benefits, anyone using such products is effectively acting as a guinea pig.

I do want to quickly survey some of the general risks to consider with the use of supplements. We are lucky to be having this discussion in a time when much more information is available regarding the safety and benefits of herbal and natural supplements than ever before. But the unknown is still a very real risk with these products. Without the regimented studies that are conducted for prescription medications, it will always be impossible to detect risks and toxicities with the same reliability. People may be experiencing a variety of side effects without realizing (or reporting) the cause – they could be considered random occurrences or could even be incorrectly pinned on another medication or supplement.

Another very real concern for which we have limited information is the possible interaction between these products and prescription medications. Drug interactions can result in increased toxicity and/or reduced benefits. For instance, if an herbal supplement were to inhibit the elimination of a prescription medication, the medication could build up to toxic levels in the body. Or, if that supplement were to induce the elimination of a prescription medication, the medication could leave the body before it even has a chance to work. St. John's Wort (typically used for depression) is the stereotypical culprit in this regard – it potently interacts with a variety of medications. In fact, there was a famous case in the 1990's in which a transplanted organ was fully rejected because the patient chose to take St. John's Wort in addition to her immunosuppressive medications, rendering them ineffective.

For those of us with gastroparesis, the gastrointestinal side effects that can occur with these products are a prominent concern. Many of them are not kind to the stomach or the intestine, and can cause stomach discomfort or pain, nausea and vomiting, indigestion, acid reflux, diarrhea, or gas. In addition to this, any number of products may interact with other medications that we need to take to maintain our health, and many of these products have also been associated with causing harm to the liver. It is important to look for these concerns when evaluating any supplement or herbal product

Anyone that takes a blood thinner (anticoagulant) is often at the greatest risk for interactions with supplements. Many products on the market can increase the risk of bleeding when taking a blood thinner, including, but not limited to:

- Bilberry
- Chamomile
- Feverfew
- Garlic
- Ginger
- Ginkgo
- Ginseng
- Grape seed
- Horse chestnut
- Red clover

that you are considering adding to your treatment regimen.

BENEFITS AND RISKS: ACUPUNCTURE

Acupuncture has been practiced for thousands of years as a Chinese remedy and is believed to have originated in Eastern cultures. It became popular in the US in the mid-1900's and has recently experienced a resurgence in popularity that is evidenced by the large number of acupuncture clinics available throughout the country.

Acupuncture is Latin for "puncture with a needle"

The basic premise of acupuncture holds that our vital energy, or Ch'i, flows through the body in the form of various channels, or meridians. These meridians, which have both a shallow and deep pathway through the body, can be blocked or imbalanced. The insertion of a needle into the skin allows for penetration of these shallow pathways and facilitates the redirection of the body's vital energy. Acupuncturists claim the ability to treat, improve, and/or cure a wide array of maladies and symptoms that can range anywhere from chronic pain, to asthma, to stomach upset.

This intervention is a great example of an alternative therapy that flummoxed scientists attempting to test its efficacy through placebo-controlled studies. How in the world do you develop a placebo treatment that mirrors the insertion of a needle into the skin? Believe it or not, someone figured it out. In fact, many methods of 'sham' acupuncture have been developed as a way to assess the placebo effect involved with acupuncture therapy!

Placebos that are used to mimic a procedure, such as a surgery, are often referred to as "sham" versions of the treatment being studied.

- Insert needles only partially

- Place the needles in locations that do not align with acupuncture doctrine

- Utilize retracting needles that do not actually enter the skin

Regardless of which technique has been used, true acupuncture has failed to show a consistent benefit

UNSUPPORTED

over sham acupuncture for the whole gamut of conditions it is claimed to treat. The only conditions for which it sometimes retains a borderline effect are nausea and vomiting and very specific types of pain, but studies have not been promising. That being said, the extent of the placebo effect that is seen with the use of acupuncture is quite impressive, and there is something to be said for the benefits and improvements that this can yield.

But benefits cannot be assessed in a void – we always have to consider the risks, too. The often exorbitant cost associated with acupuncture therapy stands out as the most real and prevalent drawback to seeking out this treatment, particularly considering its lackluster performance in placebo-controlled studies. But expense is a wholly individual decision and will differ for each person.

Acupuncture does carry some minor risks which are exactly what you might expect when needles are placed into your skin – minor pain, bleeding, bruising, faintness, and dizziness. These are mild, uncommon, and short-lived. But there are also major risks that, when they do occur on a rare basis, are significant indeed.

Viral infection spread through acupuncture needles has been documented numerous times. In fact, 35 patients in one clinic contracted hepatitis via acupuncture due to improper sterilization of needles. The owners of the clinic did not realize that simply placing needles into an alcohol bath would not kill off a virus. If you do choose to utilize acupuncture therapy, have a frank discussion with your clinic to ensure that their sterilization techniques are adequate or that new needles will be used in your sessions.

Puncture or damage to a major nerve or vital organ is the other rare but serious concern that has been reported with acupuncture. There have been isolated cases in which a needle has punctured the lungs or the heart. These are incredibly rare, but possibly fatal when they do occur. Additionally,

Risks with acupuncture

Minor:
- Pain
- Bleeding
- Bruising
- Faintness/dizziness

Major:
- Viral infection
- Organ puncture
- Nerve damage

damage to a major nerve can be an irreversible and very debilitating event. These concerns are simply important to be aware of when considering a treatment that seems to derive its benefit primarily from the placebo effect. Perhaps a discussion with your practitioner about avoiding needle placement into the chest could be helpful, as would a discussion with your doctor first about any other concerns that might be specific to your situation.

Due to the lack of evidence for benefit, acupuncture should be reserved as a last step after all medical treatments recommended by your doctor have failed. Additionally, be sure that you are not using acupuncture instead of a treatment that you know works for you. If you are fully aware of the rare but real risks involved with this therapy, you can discuss them openly with your practitioner. Ensure that steps are taken to limit the likelihood of any such issues.

BENEFITS AND RISKS: HOMEOPATHY

"Homeopathy" or "homeopathic" is an increasingly common buzzword in our culture. In fact, many people have purchased a homeopathic remedy off of the shelves at the local drugstore. Yet the average person does not fully understand what a homeopathic remedy actually is, or how it differs from any of the other treatment options surrounding it. After all, there's nothing differentiating that homeopathic fever remedy from the bottle of Tylenol sitting next to it other than the "all natural" statement on the label.

Homeopathy is Latin for "similar suffering"

Homeopathy has been around since just before 1800, and was developed by a scientist that practiced in Germany and France. The basic premise of homeopathy is purposefully counterintuitive – to treat a certain symptom, a substance that actually causes that symptom should be utilized. In order to obtain this effect, the product should be diluted down to a point at which there are no actual molecules of the original substance left.

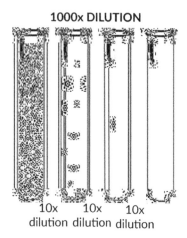

1000x DILUTION

10x dilution · 10x dilution · 10x dilution

There are also 100-fold dilution factors that are denoted with a C. For example, 1C = 100, and 2C = 20,000.

A product diluted to 30C has been diluted by a factor of:

1,000,000,000,000,000,000,000 ,000,000,000,000,000,000,000, 000,000,000,000,000,000

I seem to have some strange obsession with zeros in this book. But I'm going to take a leap here and say that this is the LARGEST string of zeros that we will ever have the opportunity to discuss, and that is not a good thing in this case!

In other words, if you are experiencing nausea, then you should consume a substance that induces nausea. However, it should be taken in homeopathic form, or a massively diluted product that ultimately contains nothing more than water. The premise of homeopathy relies on a concept called 'water memory', a concept that has yet to be proven to exist. The serial dilutions that occur to create a homeopathic product are demonstrated visually in the margin (yes, they are extensive!).

Time and time again, well-conducted placebo-controlled studies have failed to identify a benefit with the use of homeopathic remedies. This is not particularly surprising when you consider the fact that these remedies truly contain nothing more than water. In fact, the greatest concerns arise when these therapies do contain more than just water.

In recent years, we have seen an increase in the number of homeopathic therapies that actually contain a measurable quantity of the ingredient that was supposed to be diluted out. That might sound fine until you remember that the ingredients used in homeopathy will cause the symptom that you are already experiencing and attempting to alleviate.

Many examples could be provided, but I will limit the discussion to two highly representative events. In 2010, a teething tablet was found to contain belladonna, a drug that can cause seizures, difficulty breathing, excessive sleepiness, and more. And, in fact, it was causing exactly these symptoms in the babies that were receiving this product from their parents. This identical issue resurfaced in 2016, prompting the company to finally remove its teething tablet product from the market. In 2014, one of the largest recalls that occurred involved the withdrawal of 56 lots (thousands of total packages) of homeopathic products found to contain traces of penicillin. Most concerning in this situation was that the product labeling specifically stated that the products did not contain any penicillin, and this was causing severe allergic reactions in its users.

Homeopathic practitioners will identify a therapy that is most similar to the symptoms being experienced. This often results in any two homeopaths recommending very different treatments for the same ailment. Within the doctrine of homeopathy, this makes sense – multiple products can cause the same ultimate symptom and can thus be used interchangeably to treat that symptom. But what is concerning is when homeopaths recommend an unproven regimen in place of scientifically proven options. For instance, a study was conducted in which homeopaths were sought out for their recommendations regarding malaria prevention regimens for people travelling to endemic regions. These practitioners recommended homeopathic regimens in lieu of scientifically proven and universally accepted medical regimens, which has resulted in the contraction of malaria in more than one case.

A number of other homeopathic treatments have caused illness and death because they were used in place of proven medical treatments, including antibiotics and vaccines.

Again, the health risks may seem uncommon, but they are random in nature and very serious when they do occur. As there appears, time and again, to be no benefit from the use of these products, incurring any exposure to risk is very hard to justify. In addition, some of these products can be quite expensive. This expense increases dramatically when the advice of a homeopathic practitioner is sought, and that expense can pass beyond the financially tangible to include the health risks inherent in foregoing medically necessary and appropriate treatments.

#6 HARMFUL

I hope you enjoy this narrative that poignantly describes the state of the homeopathic therapy market:

Somewhere near Lyon, France, sometime this year, officials from French pharmaceutical firm Boiron will slaughter a solitary duck and extract its heart and liver - not to appease the gods but to fight the flu. The organs will be used to make an over-the-counter flu medicine, called Oscillococcinum, that will be sold around the world. In a monetary sense, this single French duck may be the most valuable *animal on the planet, as an extract of its heart and liver form the sole 'active ingredient' in a flu remedy that is expected to generate sales of $20 million or more. (For duck parts, that easily beats out foie gras in terms of return on investment.) How can Boiron claim that one duck will benefit so many sick people? Because Oscillococcinum is a homeopathic remedy, meaning that its active ingredients are so diluted that they are virtually nonexistent in the final preparation.*

– U.S. NEWS AND WORLD REPORT

OTHER ALTERNATIVE THERAPIES

We already know that there is no governmental authority regulating non-medication interventions such as surgeries and lifestyle modifications. However, the medical community studies these interventions and evaluates their benefits and risks before incorporating these treatment options into practice guidelines. This is not the case for non-medication interventions in the world of alternative therapy.

This ties back into our discussion about restrictive diets. Some of these diets have been evaluated by the medical community, and been found to be appropriate and beneficial for very specific segments of the population. For those that are appropriate, the medical community has evaluated their benefits and also become aware of the risks that may be present from following these diets. On the other hand, there are many diets out there that make nothing more than unfounded claims and may actually be dangerous to many people (see page 101). These are alternative therapies. They have not been studied and have not been placed under any level of scrutiny before their claims and popularity begin to spread like wildfire. The media and internet will tout a wide variety of lifestyle modifications, nutritional supplements, medical foods, and other exotic interventions that fall under this same umbrella – untested, unstudied alternative therapies.

The internet and bookstores run wild with every claim imaginable. If it is a remedy you seek, there is someone out there peddling it to you. I cannot stress enough the importance of considering your sources before you jump headfirst into any new ideas or therapies. Practice a regimen of common sense. If it sounds too good to be true, it likely is. If one specific therapy claims to cure all maladies known to man, how could that even be possible? And if it were, why wouldn't a drug company have snapped it up, patented it, and made billions in the process?

Be wary of anecdotal evidence. It often comes from those with the best of intentions; something worked for them and they want to share their joy with the world! More often than not, anecdotes deal in alternative therapies because they have that wild and wonderful quality – the very unknowns that attribute to their risks also make them seemingly capable of fulfilling our hopes and dreams. But that does not make any anecdote into anything more than coincidence, and it does not mean that therapy would work (or even be safe) in every other individual situation.

If there are a lot of very exciting and promising personal stories about the use of a certain therapy but you can't seem to find any studies or reputable resources that back up these claims, that should set off your Anecdote Alert!

BUT AREN'T DRUGS RISKY, TOO?

There are, without a doubt, many risks associated with FDA approved drugs. And the media loves to sensationalize them extensively. The difference is this – there appear to be many more risks with drugs only because we know so much about them. I can hand you a list of the side effects that you might experience with a medication before you start taking it. You can know how rare, common, serious, or mild these side effects are, and you can make a decision about your use of that medication. But that luxury is limited to medications only. The very thing that the media tries to vilify on a regular basis should be regarded as a gift as it enhances our ability to make informed decisions about our health.

The FDA now has a dedicated site to report adverse events caused by alternative therapies.

Reporting has gone up, but it is still done only infrequently. If you have anything to report, feel free to visit and do so! https://www.safetyreporting.hhs.gov

As awareness of concerns has grown and reporting opportunities have expanded, more and more side effects have been reported with a variety of natural and herbal products and supplements. Yet you still will not find this information included with the bottle when you pick it up from the store shelf. You will still be required to do your own research to find information about how each product could harm you.

And how did we come to know about any of these side effects at all? Because people like you and me went to the store, bought a bottle of a product that claimed to be all-natural and safe, and then fell ill. The risks of that product were not made clear, often because they were not even known. And those of us that walk away with a stomach ache or a bout of nausea are lucky in comparison to those that experience a life-threatening side effect that results in hospitalization.

I will pull no punches in my assessment of the evils of pharmaceutical companies. Too many times have there been highly publicized cases of these companies putting the wellbeing of the nation at risk in order to line their own pockets. But at least these companies have submitted themselves to some form of regulation, and they are reined in to an extent by that regulation. The corporations playing in the dietary supplement market have also found a way to lavishly line their pockets. But they have found a way to do this without concern for an agency that can rein them in when they, knowingly or unknowingly, harm the very people that are putting faith in their products.

IN SUMMARY

We have a dangerous tendency to jump to the conclusion that the term "natural" equates to good or safe. This tendency extends to our assumptions that classic or natural remedies are safer than the offerings of modern Western medicine. It is important at times such as these to conduct a reality check on our expectations. Should our hope and health be placed in the hands of a therapy that was utilized in an age when a 40-year life expectancy was acceptable and most deaths went unquestioned and undocumented? Or should more consideration be given before jumping in?

When it comes to the term medicine, there is no Eastern or Western, there is no complementary or alternative, there is either medicine that works or medicine that doesn't. And the use of alternative therapies is akin to the experience of investing in the stock market – there is a glimmer of great potential reward. But with that glimmer comes a very real and tangible level of risk.

You are ultimately the person that makes the final decision on what treatments you will and will not use. Arming yourself with the tools necessary to be an informed and critical consumer will allow you to choose only those options that are most likely to work and least likely to harm.

The potential dangers of alternative therapies:

- Possible interactions with necessary medications: Speak with a pharmacist about this possibility or utilize available resources
- Possible contamination or impurity: Utilize the resources available to protect against this
- Possibly dangerous due to unstudied risks and unreported side effects: Utilize the resources available to become fully informed
- Discouraging the use of a treatment that is actually shown to be safe and effective: Never replace proven treatments for the lofty claims of alternative therapies
- Exorbitant cost: This is an individual concern, but a very real one for many of us with a chronic condition

Personal Experience Part 7

The neurostimulator was placed. When I woke up from the surgery, I was in such excruciating pain that I couldn't breathe. It turns out that when they cut through your abdominal wall (solid muscle!), stick something through it (the leads), and then place something bulky inside of it (the device), your body doesn't react very well. The recovery nurse was desperately trying to give me pain medications to help me breathe, but with no luck. Clasping a pillow against my stomach helped, but I was still struggling to take in air. Then the surgeon came over and said something to the nurse. She gave me two drugs and the pain dissolved. During that night in the hospital, I stayed hooked up to a pain medication and felt more than capable of dealing with the much more tolerable pain in my stomach.

The next day, I insisted on going home. The doctor prescribed some oral narcotics and ibuprofen. I was soon to discover that I do not tolerate oral narcotics well - they make me very nauseated and I vomit them right back up. So my pain medication for the remainder of my recovery was limited to ibuprofen. Not the strongest or the greatest, but oh well - this was a small hurdle compared to the ones I had already been dealt!

Besides the persistent pain, I soon began to experience the muscle tissue spasming around my new device. It was so uncomfortable that I called the surgeon on-call overnight and asked for a muscle relaxant. Much to my delight, that muscle relaxant not only calmed the spasm but also made me very sleepy for the first few nights. A welcomed relief!

For the first few weeks I was unable to sleep in any position other than on my back with my knees bent. My iron deficiency had become so bad (not helped by the blood loss from the surgery) that I had developed persistent restless leg syndrome. Many people don't realize that this is actually a relatively common result of iron deficiency. Restless leg syndrome causes your legs to kick in your sleep, and for some people, this can wake them up. It disrupts sleep cycles and causes a lot of fatigue, which is then only compounded by the fatigue caused by the iron deficiency that brought this on in the first place. I was placed on iron supplements, and we will talk more about those later.

It was also over 6 weeks before I was able to stand up straight and walk upright after my surgery. Prior to that I was slightly hunched over due to the healing and rebuilding occurring in my abdomen. Lifting anything that was more than a few pounds during this time was also out of the question, as it led to a lot of pain and convinced me that I would certainly rip out my stitches and cause the stimulator to fall right out!

The biggest change that I experienced immediately post-surgery, however, was the swelling in my stomach. I looked at least 4-5 months pregnant for the first few months after surgery. And that swelling was not only pushing out my belly, it was also pressing in on my stomach. My meal sizes shrank drastically. I was lucky to be able to eat a piece of toast with an egg before I started to feel a lot of pain and pressure. The unexpected advantage to this was that it trained me in portion size restriction (which I will be the first to admit I have always struggled with because I love food).

And then something truly wonderful happened a few weeks after the surgery - I felt hungry! At first, I had no idea what it was. I thought it was some foreboding new signal from my stomach that something was wrong. And then when I ate something, it went away. The next time it happened a few days later, it finally dawned on me. I was feeling hungry again for the first time in 6 years. It still doesn't occur often, but I am incredibly grateful every time that it does. I never thought I could savor something that I had previously considered an uncomfortable nuisance, but here we are. The old adage to appreciate the small things takes on a new meaning after you've experienced the peaks and valleys of a chronic condition like gastroparesis.

It took almost an entire year after placement of the stimulator for me to be fully back to myself. I was swollen for quite some time after and experienced various pains and spasms in that area as the scar tissue slowly resolved. A few times, even into the second year, I was in so much pain that I had to go to the emergency room to ensure that nothing was malfunctioning - no leads were disconnected or wrapped around my intestines. Thankfully, no severe complications like that ever occurred for me. And eventually the severe pains, mild pains, and spasms subsided. I just had this oblong metal object sitting quietly under my skin. Sometimes it would remind me of its presence by jiggling around like a jumping bean, and then it would quiet itself down again.

Nutritional Supplementation

10

"I am not afraid of storms for I am learning how to sail my ship."

LOUISA MAY ALCOTT

Now that we have had discussions about both dietary supplements and restrictive diets, we get to take a quick trip through a territory that combines both topics – nutritional supplementation.

NUTRIENT DEFICIENCY

We only need to supplement our nutrition when we have a deficiency of some type. A nutrient deficiency indicates that the body is low in a particular substance that is important to cell or organ function. In the case of vitamins and minerals, these substances are referred to as micronutrients and are not produced by the body, so they must be consumed in our diets. The complications of nutrient deficiencies typically become worse over time, although some can be immediately noticeable.

Macronutrients:
Proteins, carbohydrates, fats

Micronutrients:
Vitamins and minerals

As you have seen throughout my personal story, I have experienced points in my life in which I was deficient in a number of crucial nutrients. This state is in no way isolated to me – nutrient deficiencies are quite common in people with GI conditions of any type. Those with gastroparesis are likely to be deficient in nutrients for a couple of different reasons, the primary one being a limited and constrained diet. In fact, those of us with gastroparesis are more likely to experience deficiencies earlier on in our journeys because this typically represents the time frame in which our diets are the most poorly managed.

Another reason that those with gastroparesis can become deficient in nutrients is due to poor absorption of the ones that are consumed. You'll remember in our discussion of medications in the GI tract that the intestine can only absorb certain medications in certain environments, and that foods and nutrients may compete for absorption (see page 55). For those whose emptying is significantly delayed, exceptional competition can begin to occur in which various foods and substances come together to lend to a poor environment for nutrient absorption.

This is markedly different than the poor absorption seen as a result of intestinal damage in conditions such as celiac disease or IBD. The reasons for poor absorption with gastroparesis provide us with more control over improving our nutritional status.

Intestinal damage from an inflammatory condition must be allowed to heal and repair in order to return to a more normal state of absorption.

It may seem daunting at first to ensure that you are obtaining appropriate nutrition. In fact, you may hear from people that taking vitamin X or mineral Y really helped them with Z, but that has nothing to do with a nutrient deficiency. A deficiency will result in complications if it continues, and it must be addressed for the sake of your immediate and long-term health. There is a great way to filter out the noise and find a place to start – request a blood test. Your doctor can order the appropriate panel to look for deficiencies in nutrients that are typically obtained through the diet. This will paint a clear picture for where you are starting out and where you need to be.

It can be tempting to just start adding supplements across the board, but instead you should try to focus on only those nutrients where you are truly deficient.

A number of large studies have recently been published that have shown that it is not beneficial to take supplements without a deficiency and in some cases may actually be harmful.

HOW TO SUPPLEMENT NUTRIENTS

I will start off with a very clear statement:

If there is an opportunity to obtain a nutrient through your diet, this is far superior to any other forms of supplementation

It may initially seem that the most straightforward and manageable way to address a nutrient deficiency is to take a supplement for that nutrient. But let's break down the reasons that this is not actually the case.

1. **Pill burden**

   I'm sure you would be upset to discover that your elderly relative had been unknowingly taking a Vitamin C supplement every day instead of his blood pressure medication, landing him in the hospital.

   Believe it or not, these are actually common occurrences and a very real reason to eliminate unnecessary pills.

   This is a term used to describe the impact that the number of medications and supplements that must be taken can have on a person's ability to take them. For instance, if you find that you need to supplement 3 nutrients and you are already taking 4 medications, that means that you have to take around 7-14 pills a day, depending. For some people, this may become difficult to remember. For others, it is simply tedious. My entire career is built around medication, and I will openly admit to my tendency to stray from what I am supposed to be taking when the number or frequency gets too high. It's just human nature and no one enjoys taking pills (or drinking poor-tasting liquids).

2. **Side effects**

   Just as with medications, supplements can cause side effects. They are different for each product, but not surprisingly, they almost all occur in the GI tract. Whether it be nausea, stomach pain, constipation, or diarrhea, none of these are side effects that those of us with gastroparesis want to add to our current situations. If the supplement tablet causes nausea but you can eat that nutrient in your diet without any issues, wouldn't that be preferred?

3. **Absorption**

   Believe it or not, your body often absorbs nutrients better when they are a part of a natural food product than when they are in a concentrated supplement form. Although the science isn't fully understood in every case, there are many examples of 'food synergy' in which the valuable nutrients found in a product such as a fruit or vegetable are more happily absorbed than in a tablet form.

4. **Sustainability**

Identifying foods which you are able to tolerate that contain the nutrient that you need will help you in expanding your diet. It is also guaranteed to bring more nutrients along with it, since foods always contain multiple nutrients. Being able to obtain that nutrient from your food and not from a supplement protects you from a variety of issues, including days in which you are not able to keep down any tablets that you swallow, or affordability issues with obtaining a certain supplement.

All of these points considered, let's spend a little bit of time talking about the nuances of obtaining nutrients through our diets before we talk about specific nutrients or the supplements that can be used to correct deficiencies.

THE NUTRITIONAL VALUE OF FOODS

As a pharmacist, I have been trained in nutrient deficiencies and how to treat them, and have gained plenty of experience in this area as I've practiced. However, I think that a brief discussion of dietary considerations is incredibly important before we discuss supplements. As I am not a trained dietician, my room to speak on this subject is limited, so we will keep to a very specific focus – the nutritional value of the foods that we eat.

PROCESSED AND WHOLE FOODS

Although this is a topic worthy of its own book , we should briefly discuss the quality of the foods that we choose to eat. We live in a society in which most of the foods that we have access to are processed. And in fact, we've become so desensitized to it that we don't necessarily even notice when it has happened. For instance, you might make cookies at

I would highly recommend a book that does already exist on this topic - In Defense of Food by Michael Pollan. This is a wonderful introduction to the nutritional value of whole versus processed foods from a very talented author whose books are evidence-based.

home and use about 8-10 ingredients. So then why is it that the cookies you are purchasing from the store have an ingredient list so long it practically falls off of the package? And why aren't we able to recognize half of those ingredient names?

The term "whole foods" here is not in reference to the grocery store chain. It implies foods that are in their natural form – full fruits and vegetables, eggs, meats, grains, etc. These contain complexes of micronutrients and macronutrients as they were produced in nature. While it is true (and very important) that the nutritive value of each of these items can also vary, that is again the topic for a different book and one best left to experts in that field.

Another example of processed foods are foods that come in forms that wouldn't be possible without significant manipulation and chemical additives. For instance, margarine is made of vegetable fat, which is a liquid at room temperature. In order to develop a substance that would remain solid at room temperature, food scientists performed

chemical reactions that created trans-fats. Many of you are likely familiar with this term due to all of the negative publicity it received when it was realized that it may be detrimental to our health. This was particularly upsetting because margarine was developed as a healthier alternative to butter. In fact, many of the foods that are developed to be compliant with a specific diet are highly processed. This is particularly true of gluten-free items which contain extra sugar, fat, and additives to obtain the desired consistency and flavor in the absence of wheat flour.

Other examples of processed products include milk made from almonds or soy, which requires additives to obtain the desired texture. Carrageenan is commonly found in these products and has been associated with GI upset. Similarly, many of the juices that you will find in the store contain very little of the actual fruit on the label and large amounts of sugar or flavorings instead.

One advantage of processed foods is that many have been fortified with additional nutrients. For instance, cereals are typically packed full of B vitamins. Those almond and soy milks are chock full of calcium. Those juices are infused with vitamin C. But do you notice a common theme? Many of these products are simply fortifying themselves with the nutrients that were eliminated when they were processed. And as we will discuss next, the body does a better job of absorbing nutrients when they are naturally contained in a whole food product, as opposed to when they are added after the fact.

FOOD SYNERGY

I had mentioned previously that although we do not always understand why, it appears that our bodies are more able to absorb nutrients from foods than from supplements. We are also aware of food combinations that allow our bodies to better absorb some of the valuable nutrients that are present.

Some studies have been conducted that have directly compared the consumption of a specific nutrient from food to the consumption of that nutrient from a pill. These studies have consistently shown that the levels of that nutrient in the body increase more rapidly when obtained from the food than from the supplement. This may not be true for all products, and we don't necessarily have a scientific explanation for why this happens, but it is likely related to components of the food that make the nutrient more compatible with the tissues in our intestine.

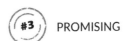 PROMISING

Let's take a look at a few specific examples of how these properties can be used to help us improve our nutrient intake through our diets.

EXAMPLE 1: IRON

Iron supplements must be taken two to three times a day for many weeks before iron returns to the appropriate level in the body. From then on, iron must be taken daily to continue to maintain these levels. These supplements are notorious for causing nausea, stomach pain, and significant constipation.

Best source of iron:
Meat

Less ideal sources:
Plant products and supplements

Iron absorption enhancer:
Vitamin C

Iron absorption is very poor when it is obtained from plant products and supplements. However, its absorption more than doubles when it is obtained from meat products. We know that this happens because the iron comes in an enveloped form that is quickly sucked up by the intestine. Consistent intake of small amounts of iron-rich meats (such as red meats) can allow for iron maintenance or replenishment at a more rapid rate than through the use of supplements.

Attempts to obtain adequate iron intake from plant products can be frustrating due to the 50% reduction in absorption. However, if meat is out of the question for any reason, it is still easier on the GI tract than the use of supplements. Certain plant products are higher in iron than others. Additionally, vitamin C can increase iron absorption significantly, especially through the diet. So what about adding juice or fruit to your meal?

EXAMPLE 2: VITAMIN D

Vitamin D supplements are popular and widely available. They are usually taken once a day to maintain adequate vitamin D levels. These supplements are known to cause nausea, vomiting, and stomach pain.

Best source of vitamin D:
Sunlight

Less ideal sources:
Fish skin, oils, and supplements

Vitamin D absorption enhancer:
Fats

The best way to obtain Vitamin D is actually through sun exposure. In fact, for a person with light skin, very minimal amounts of sun exposure will stimulate adequate production of Vitamin D in the body. This exposure is typically less than what usually triggers us to apply sunscreen. For instance, the average person (recognizing that there are many interacting factors such as altitude, cloud cover, skin color, etc) can receive adequate exposure to only the arms, face, or legs over just 15 minutes, twice a week. Of course, skin cancer is a concern that is ever-present, so each person must consider their own risks and lifestyle.

Vitamin D is not present in many natural food products, but it is highly concentrated in fish skins and oils. It is also already added to many of our dairy products, including milk, butter, and yogurt. Although this is not ideal, the fortification of your food products is probably enough to prevent you from needing a separate supplement as well.

EXAMPLE 3: VITAMINS A, E, AND K

Although deficiencies in these three vitamins are very rare, they are usually available as supplements in tablets or capsules. These supplements are unusual in that they are not often associated with many side effects when taken, but high doses can cause toxicity.

These vitamins are all fat-soluble, which means that they dissolve in fat. It also means that they collect in the fat tissues within our bodies. This fat solubility can be used to our advantage and help us to eliminate the need to take these as additional pills because these vitamins are absorbed more rapidly by our bodies when they are eaten with fatty foods. For instance, when eating green, leafy vegetables, utilizing a dressing that contains some fat can allow for great absorption of these nutrients.

Best source of vitamin A, E, K: Foods with higher fat content

Less ideal sources: Supplements

Vitamin absorption enhancer: Fats

NUTRIENT OVERVIEW

The below represents the micronutrients that are most often discussed in relation to a GI condition. This list is not meant to be complete or encompass every possible consideration. The information found here should help to build a foundational understanding for the roles that a variety of micronutrients can play in our bodies and the unique considerations that must be made for each one.

CALCIUM

What is it? A mineral that plays a crucial role in nerve activity, muscle movement, and bone formation

Other names: Its elemental abbreviation – Ca

Deficiencies can cause: Muscle cramps, confusion, depression, and stiff, sore muscles. Low calcium levels over an extended time can lend to bone issues, such as osteoporosis.

Sources: Dairy products, kale, broccoli, calcium-set tofu

Can you have too much? The body needs to maintain a certain range of calcium in the body, and too much is just as bad as too little. When calcium levels become high, it can build up in the body and collect, causing problems like kidney stones and possibly even heart and blood vessel issues.

Your body is only able to take in so much calcium at once, which is why most calcium supplements say to take them twice a day.

It is when your body tries to get rid of extra calcium through the urine that it can run into issues like kidney stones. It is best not to take more than 500mg of calcium in one dose.

IRON

What is it? A metal responsible for carrying oxygen through the blood along with something called hemoglobin

Other names: Ferrous, ferric, or its elemental abbreviation – Fe

Deficiencies can cause: Reduced oxygen circulation and anemia, which can lead to severe fatigue

Sources: Meats, fruits, vegetables

Can you have too much? Extra iron that is taken by mouth will be discarded by the body, so there is no toxicity from buildup over time. Taking too much at one time can cause a lot of GI discomfort.

If you ever hear of iron overload, it typically refers to a build-up of iron from IV supplementation or from receiving a lot of blood transfusions for a long time.

Iron toxicity can occur in small children that consume large quantities at once through an accidental exposure.

MAGNESIUM

What is it? An abundant substance that is involved in working with many enzymes in our bodies

Other names: Its elemental abbreviation – Mg

Deficiencies can cause: Minor deficiencies do not cause many symptoms, and may result in fatigue or weight loss. Very significant deficiency can cause nausea, muscle cramps, and seizures.

Sources: Green, leafy vegetables, whole grains, nuts, meats, milk

Can you have too much? Any extra magnesium will be eliminated from the body through the urine, so there is no concern for magnesium toxicity over time. Taking too much magnesium at once, though, typically results in severe diarrhea.

We will actually talk about how magnesium is purposely used for this exact reason in the second part of the book.

POTASSIUM

What is it? This is an electrolyte, which means that it is important for maintaining the volume of fluid in our blood and in our cells, as well as playing an important role in nerve activity

Other names: Its elemental abbreviation – K

Deficiencies can cause: Deficiencies in potassium are actually typically due to losing too much from diarrhea or vomiting as opposed to not consuming enough. Deficiencies can cause muscle weakness and muscle disorders that worsen in severity as the potassium level drops.

Sources: Fruits and vegetables, dairy, meats, nuts

Can you have too much? The body will eliminate additional potassium through the urine, particularly when in the doses that can be found from supplements or food.

VITAMIN A

What is it? This vitamin is crucial to various bodily processes

Other names: Retinol. You may also hear of members of this family referred to as the carotenes or carotenoids. These are considered 'precursors' of the vitamin A that is used in the body.

Precursor:

An inactive molecule that is converted into an active form

Deficiencies can cause: Poor vision and immune function, skin conditions

Sources: Dairy products, fish, darkly colored fruits, leafy vegetables

This is an interesting one. While Vitamin A itself is fat-soluble, the carotenes (precursors for vitamin A) are actually water-soluble. That means that if you are taking a carotene, you do not need to worry about it building up and causing toxicity the way that Vitamin A does.

What is the result of taking too much carotene? Orange skin!

Can you have too much? As a fat-soluble vitamin, A can build up in the body over time. Too much of this vitamin can cause toxicity, often in the liver.

VITAMIN B (1-12)

What is it? A family of vitamins that, while they each have their own distinct function in the body, are typically crucial components in the production of fats and proteins and in metabolism.

Other Names: This category includes thiamine (B1), riboflavin (B2), niacin (B3), pyridoxine (B6), biotin (B7), folic acid (B9), cyanocobalamin (B12), and more.

Deficiencies can cause: Deficiencies in these substances can have notable short- and long-term impacts on the body, from hair loss and fatigue to nerve pain and fetal development issues.

Sources: Although they are different for each specific B vitamin, they can generally be found in whole grains, enriched food products (such as cereals), dark leafy vegetables, and some meats

Can you have too much? In a typical situation, no. These vitamins are water-soluble, which means that we get rid of the extra in our urine. However, this also means that taking huge doses of any of these does not help – all of that extra ends up leaving the body.

VITAMIN C

This deficiency is also the cause of scurvy! The discovery that citrus fruit could prevent scurvy was one of the first examples of modern medicine identifying a cause and effect. Imagine how mind-boggling such a discovery must have been before nutrients were understood.

It is important to note that Vitamin C levels cannot be tested in the blood and a deficiency is rarely a concern in modern civilization.

What is it? This vitamin is crucial to a lot of processes in the body and is also an antioxidant that helps to neutralize harmful molecules.

Other Names: Ascorbic acid, ascorbate (a popular component in cold remedies that, in case you were wondering, the evidence does not support)

Deficiencies can cause: Deficiencies in vitamin C are rare but can slowly develop into weakness, irritability, weight loss and muscle and nerve pain.

Sources: Citrus fruit, strawberries, tomatoes, spinach, Brussel sprouts, cauliflower

Can you have too much? In a typical situation, no. Vitamin C is water-soluble, which means that we get rid of the extra in our urine. However, large doses of Vitamin C can cause a lot of stomach upset, nausea, and diarrhea.

VITAMIN D

What is it? This vitamin is responsible for helping to regulate our calcium and phosphorous levels, which contributes to our bone health

Other names: Cholecalciferol (D3), ergocalciferol (D2)

Deficiencies can cause: This has been associated with a number of possible issues, including osteoporosis, heart health, and more. However, these concerns are still limited to association only – cause and effect has been difficult to confirm (see page 19).

Sources: Fish oils, egg yolks, exposure to the sun

Can you have too much? As a fat-soluble vitamin, D can build up in the body and cause toxicity when levels become too high. Toxicity can lead to kidney and heart issues.

VITAMIN E

What is it? This vitamin is an important antioxidant that helps to neutralize harmful molecules

Other names: a-tocopherol

Deficiencies can cause: This is most commonly only a concern in children who require a store of this vitamin for appropriate vision and nerve function.

Sources: Nuts, fruits, vegetable oils, whole grains

Can you have too much? As a fat-soluble vitamin, E can build up in the body and cause toxicity when levels become too high. This has not been reported often, but may include severe bleeding and stroke. In addition, some studies have indicated that taking more vitamin E than needed over an extended period of time may increase overall risk of death. It is important to note that if anyone has a known issue with their kidneys that results in reduced function, they can be at an increased risk for developing high levels of nutrients that might normally be removed from the body through the urine. This typically only happens when kidney function is severely impaired, but it is an important consideration for a small subset of people.

You may be wondering about other commonly discussed nutrients, such as selenium, chromium phosphorous, zinc, manganese, iodine, etc. The reason that I did not include these here is that deficiencies are exceptionally rare, particularly in developed countries. Many of these may be the subject of articles and blogs claiming that deficiencies in these products are the cause of many of our health complaints. Science has been unable to validate these claims and regular supplementation is typically not recommended or helpful.

NUTRITIONAL SUPPLEMENTS

The ideal will always be to obtain your nutrients from your diet. Ensure that you are eating high-quality foods that allow for the highest nutritional value. Attempt to vary your diet by specifically identifying foods that contain the nutrient that you need and finding one that is tolerable for you. Even just taking in small amounts of a food (such as bites of meat) can go a lot further than you might expect.

If supplementing through the diet is simply not possible, either because the deficiency is too large or your diet is too restrictive, then supplements are available that can help to treat these deficiencies. One of the points that I made in our discussion on alternative therapies is that vitamins and minerals are actually considered to be dietary supplements (see page 114). This relegates them to that class of products that are not subject to the FDA regulation that we expect. Fortunately, most vitamins and minerals can be found from a company that has obtained third-party certification of its products, allowing you to protect yourself from any harm related to poor quality or manufacturing (see page

As I'm sure you are aware, the internet abounds with anecdotes regarding the micronutrients and trace minerals that are causing all of our problems. However, this is a well-studied field and those claims have not been validated.

Please be particularly careful when searching for information on nutrient deficiencies online. Many of the websites that appear are sponsored by companies that make supplements and even more are rife with anecdotal and crazy claims. Try to limit yourself to medical references and government-based dietary and nutrition sites.

119). As long as we start there, we can focus on the pros and cons of the supplements themselves.

Be wary of supplements that have mega doses of their ingredients. You can identify these if the bottle states that the ingredient provides >200% of the recommended daily intake. This is never necessary and can sometimes be harmful if an ingredient builds up in the body. Additionally, mega doses are more likely to cause stomach and GI upset, something that we always like to avoid.

It is also helpful to pay attention to the form of the supplement that you are taking. You will notice that many of the products that you see on the shelf will have a different second name. For instance, you can buy iron as iron sulfate or iron gluconate and calcium as calcium carbonate and calcium citrate. Each of these forms can cause different side effects (constipation vs diarrhea) and will be absorbed differently (better with or without food).

NUTRITIONAL SUPPLEMENTATION RESOURCE

The US government has a wonderful resource on the National Institutes of Health (NIH) website that will help you to break down the attributes of your supplement options. I highly recommend visiting this website if you ever have any questions regarding nutrient deficiencies and how to supplement, either through the diet or through supplements. This resource provides guidance on which foods can be helpful for supplementation and how much is needed on a daily basis. It also discusses the different forms of each supplement and their pros and cons. All-in-all, it is a wonderful resource that I believe is superior to anything that I could offer here, and it will be continuously updated online. Through the topics and concepts discussed here, you now have the understanding and resources needed to actively manage your care in relation to diagnosed deficiencies or suggestions that you receive regarding nutrients.

https://ods.od.nih.gov/factsheets/

Select the Consumer Sheet, which provides a complete summary of the information that you need in order to make an educated choice.

Personal Experience

It was very difficult to notice any changes in my symptoms during that first year due to the swelling, pain, and constricted stomach volume. When I went in for a checkup at about 6 months, the doctor discovered that there was a lot of resistance and he increased the settings of my stimulator to a much higher level so that the electrical stimulation could push through to my stomach. As the swelling disappeared and I was able to take in slightly larger quantities of food, I began paying very close attention to my lifestyle again. I focused on eating the right foods, at the right times, in the right quantities. I fell back into my heavy walking habit to ensure that I was getting good activity. And I continued to drink carbonated water with a splash of fruit juice.

Once I had all of this back in place, I really assessed the nutritional status of my diet. I started to add in different forms of some of the items that I could eat, to provide a broader range of nutrients. I also decided that now that I had things slightly more under control, I could try adding back tiny amounts of items that would greatly benefit me nutritionally. For instance, I was unable to eat meat (or at least thought that I was), and eliminated it completely from my diet. However, this left me iron deficient and low in protein. After some experimenting with iron-rich meats, I discovered that I could eat small bites of sausage each day without experiencing a negative impact. Not only was this a delicious discovery, it was also of enormous benefit to my body. A handful of similar changes made an exceptional difference for my health.

I began to gain back my weight. My skin took its color back. I went to the doctor and my labs were normal for the first time in years. I felt capable of walking further, and even starting going on hikes. I was less frightened of my symptoms getting in the way of my daily life. I still had my constant regurgitation of food throughout the day, and I still had plenty of bouts of nausea, dizziness, stomach pain, gas, and bloating, but it was all reduced to a more tolerable amount. I could live like this. In fact, I knew that I could live well like this.

Alternative Nutrition Methods

11

We have spent the entirety of the first section of this book discussing the many foundational concepts that are necessary to understand the GI tract, gastroparesis, and the treatment options that are so often presented to us. I want to wrap up this section by discussing what happens when you are not able to handle eating your foods at all, no matter how many accommodations and changes you make. In this case, alternative methods for obtaining your nutrition must be explored.

Don't forget that we have yet to discuss specific topics that can aid in gastroparesis management and help to keep the symptoms in check!

Most people will not find themselves in this situation, and the use of alternative options for obtaining one's food should be reserved only for people with very severe, persistent symptoms. The use of alternative methods should not be jumped into without careful consideration, and they should rarely be viewed as a permanent solution. We will discuss the pros and cons to these options here, building on everything that we have learned thus far in this section.

FEEDING TUBES

The purpose for using a feeding tube in gastroparesis is to bypass the stomach and deliver nutrition directly to the intestine. This means that the paralysis of the stomach has become so severe that the symptoms associated with eating cannot be tolerated. In order to ensure that a person maintains adequate nutrition, they must receive it through a tube that can place those nutrients into the intestine for absorption.

Feeding tubes are used for a variety of other reasons as well, and as such they come in various types that are either permanent or temporary in nature. I am going to cover all of the terms that you might run into, even though they will not all be used for gastroparesis.

Nasogastric (NG) Tube: A temporary tube that is placed down the nose and into the stomach. This is typically used at times when a person is not able to swallow their medications on their own.

Gastrostomy (G) Tube: A permanent tube that is surgically placed into the stomach through the abdomen. This tube can be accessed from a point on the abdomen. It is typically used for people that are not able to swallow their foods, or for people that need help keeping up with their nutritional requirements in addition to the foods that they eat.

Nasoduodenal (ND) Tube: A temporary tube that is placed down the nose and into the duodenum. This is typically used at times when a person is experiencing extreme nausea or vomiting and simply needs to bypass their stomach for the time being.

Nasojejunal (NJ) Tube: A temporary tube that is placed down the nose and into the jejunum. This may be used in the same situations as a naso-duodenal tube, and is also often used as a test for whether or not a person can tolerate nutrition entering the jejunum directly.

Jejunostomy (J) Tube: A permanent tube that is surgically placed into the jejunum through the abdomen. This tube can be accessed from a point on the abdomen. A nasojejunal tube may be used as a test to make sure someone can tolerate foods entering the jejunum directly prior to the placement of this tube. This is the tube that is used for people that cannot tolerate foods entering the stomach for extended durations of time.

As you can imagine from reading these descriptions, a person with gastroparesis is most likely to utilize an ND or NJ tube when they are experiencing a temporary but very severe increase in symptoms. For symptoms that are permanently preventing someone from being able to eat their foods, a J-tube will provide a longer term solution to this problem.

If you think back to our discussion of the GI tract, you might be wondering why it is preferred to send food directly to the jejunum instead of the duodenum (see page 33). Interestingly, placing nutrition directly into the duodenum seems to stimulate a lot of secretions from the pancreas that are not needed and may cause GI side effects. Additionally, food that is placed into the duodenum sometimes has a tendency to reflux back into the stomach through the pyloric sphincter. Skipping over the duodenum and going directly to the jejunum eliminates both of these concerns.

J-Tubes bypass:
- Mouth
- Esophagus
- Esophageal sphincter
- Stomach
- Pyloric sphincter
- Duodenum

J-Tube feeds pass through:
- Jejunum
- Ileum
- Large intestine (colon)

TUBE PLACEMENT

Nasal tubes are placed by sliding the tube down the nose and into the GI tract. In certain situations, a tiny camera may be inserted into the nose along with the tube, allowing the physician to see where the tube is going within the GI tract. It is very important to be certain that the tube is placed into the desired area, so if a camera cannot be placed down the nose, the doctor may actually conduct an endoscopy. There are also other methods available that are used at different clinics and hospitals, including the use of radiology to identify the final location of the tube.

Jejunostomy tubes are placed surgically, and people are usually placed under anesthesia for the placement of the tube. A hole is cut into the abdomen and through the stomach, where the tip of the tube is then pushed through to the desired part of the GI tract, which for a J-tube, would be the jejunum. The placement of this tube is usually evaluated through an endoscopy or even a colonoscopy, which makes sense because the person is already asleep for the procedure.

FEEDING THROUGH A TUBE

I am sure that many of you have already reached the conclusion that the food that is placed into a tube must be liquid. This is obviously necessary because the tube itself must remain unclogged, which means that a liquid must be used instead of solids or powders. But it is also necessary because the mechanical and chemical digestion that happens in the stomach is being bypassed (see page 29). This means that the food that enters the jejunum must also be basically digested and ready for absorption by the intestines.

Nutritional formulas specifically prepared for J-Tube use are:

- Pre-digested
- "A complete diet"
- Deplete of flavorings

There are a number of medical nutrition products that are made specifically for use in a J-tube. These products are formulas that contain the basic macro and micro nutrients that are required for adequate nutrition. Because taste is not a concern, these formulas do not contain any additives or unnecessary sugars to improve the flavor of the product. However, due to our incomplete understanding for food synergy and all of the concepts that play into overall nutrition, the body does miss out on many of the benefits of eating whole foods (see page 143).

As far as practicality goes, the intestine represents a much more constricted space than your stomach. We are used to being able to pour large quantities of liquids and solids down our throats because the stomach is a bit like a bowl that everything just drops into. In fact, it even tries to accommodate us when we go really crazy by expanding. The intestine, on the other hand, is a narrow, long tube with no bowl at the end. You obviously can't feasibly sit there and slowly pour liquids into a hole in your abdomen. Instead, J–Tube feeds are administered on a pump. This allows for the formula to be pumped at a steady rate into the intestine. In order to avoid sugar imbalances and the fainting, sweating, and more that can come with them, the pumps run over hours at a time.

The jejunum has very specific expectations for the items that enter it, and anything that does not meet these expectations can lead to diarrhea, pain, and cramping. Multiple factors must be considered in order to make these feeds as comfortable as possible for the person receiving them. The speed at which the formula is given and the total length of time over which it is given can be tweaked on the pump to improve tolerability. It might also be necessary to try different types of formula to find one that is more acceptable to your intestine. In short, J–tube feeds are not without their own discomforts, and they will need to be monitored and altered to find the right approach for each person.

RISKS

It is also important to recognize that feeding tubes come with a number of risks and obstacles. We have already mentioned some of these in relation to the careful tweaking that must be done to minimize the side effects caused by J–tube feeds. In addition, there are some frustrating complications that might occur with these tubes, including infection and irritation at the J–tube insertion site on the abdomen. This can be the reason for a number of visits to the doctor and a lot of discomfort.

Risks with J-Tube use:

- Intolerance of feeds
- Infection
- Skin irritation
- Dislocation
- Clogging
- Leaking

The tubes also tend to malfunction and fall out of place. Malfunctions include situations in which the tube becomes clogged and cannot be used to administer formulas until it is unclogged. There are also times when the tube begins to leak. Besides being messy and inconvenient, significant leaking can lead to questions regarding how much of the nutrition you actually received. One of the more common risks with these tubes is their tendency to fall out of place. This means that the part of the tube that is supposed to be in the jejunum actually migrates to a different part of the intestine, which can cause discomfort with feeds and alter absorption.

Another consideration with the use of J-tube feeds is whether or not you are eating anything at all or are receiving all of your intake through the tube. In order for your stomach to maintain its functionality, it is always best to try to keep taking in small amounts of food. This is also important for possible future efforts to return to receiving nutrition through eating. Additionally, your stomach will continue to produce acid whether or not you are eating. Thus, people who receive their nutrition through J-tube feeds often experience a lot of acid reflux. We will discuss this topic further in the next section of the book.

For all of the reasons that we have just discussed, every effort should always be made to return to obtaining your nutrition by eating. Feeding tubes are a necessary option for people who are struggling to maintain their nutritional status, but they are a far less than ideal option for permanent use. In the next section of the book we will discuss many of the considerations that can be made in managing our conditions, as well as other treatment options, such as the neurostimulator. All of that being said, I do realize that permanent feeding tube use will be necessary for a small number of people.

MEDICATIONS AND FEEDING TUBES

We have spent plenty of time talking about the ways that medications and the GI tract interact. You can imagine that placing medications through feeding tubes and directly into the jejunum might disrupt some of the concepts that we've already discussed.

I don't want to go into too much detail on this topic, but I do think that there are some main points that should be covered and that each person with a feeding tube should be aware of, so I will list them here.

1. Tablets and capsules will always need to be altered in order to be placed into a feeding tube. The same Do Not Crush List that we discussed previously should be used in these situations (see page 64). If a medication is on this list, you must either swallow it by mouth or talk to your doctor about your options.

2. Some liquid versions of medications actually bind to feeding tubes, preventing them from working and also often causing clogs. Speak with your pharmacist to make sure that any of the products that are you are taking do not have this problem.

3. You will remember in our discussion that medications are absorbed in different parts of the GI tract depending on their preferences, and not all are absorbed in the jejunum. This means that if given through a J-tube, some drugs may not work as well because they are not fully absorbed and other drugs might cause extra side effects because more is absorbed.

   We do not always have good information on when this might happen. It is important for you to know that this is a concern and to try to take medications by mouth whenever possible. If you must place it through the J-tube, be vigilant for changes in the impact of the medication, whether that it doesn't work as well or it causes increased side effects.

4. Some medications may bind to or compete with the formula that you are getting through the J-tube, making them difficult to absorb. This can be hard to avoid because J-tube feeds are given so often throughout the day. If possible, take the medications by mouth or through the tube when feeds are not running. Otherwise, be vigilant for changes in the way that the drug works.

If you are on a number of medications and also have a J-tube, you should have a conversation with your doctor about the issues that I have listed here. It is always a good idea to make sure that everyone on your team is aware of potential issues and that you are all working together to ensure that your health is managed in the best possible way.

IV NUTRITION

I am going to keep this section very brief because IV (intravenous) nutrition is such a highly undesirable option for long-term use and rarely considered for people with gastroparesis. Feeding tubes will almost always be the appropriate option for cases in which the stomach is simply not functional. However, in situations where the entire GI tract has become unusable for some reason (such as a blockage), IV nutrition may be considered as a way to maintain nutritional status and allow the GI tract to rest temporarily.

IV nutrition must be prepared in a sterile manufacturing location and then delivered to your home, at which point it is administered continuously over the majority of the day. This is both an expensive and inconvenient option that inhibits many daily living activities. In order to receive IV nutrition, an IV line or port must be placed, which carries with it a number of risks, including the risk of a blood stream infection. Additionally, the use of IV nutrition in the long-term can lead to significant complications for the GI tract and the liver. Whenever possible, IV nutrition should be avoided or only considered as a short-term solution.

Part II

The first part of this book was spent building a strong foundation in the con-cepts necessary to truly understand gastroparesis and the many factors that can impact symptoms and nutrition. With the transition into Part II, we will break down the details and considerations in the treatment for gastroparesis and its associated conditions. It is very important that I reiterate the need to discuss any ideas and treatment changes with a medical provider that is familiar with you. While the information in this book may be pertinent and useful to you, it should not be implemented without medical advice from a medical professional that knows your situation.

We will focus primarily on medications, although we will also discuss non-medication prevention and treatment options as well. Special care was taken to make sure that the most pertinent issues related to gastroparesis remain the primary focus of this section. There are a number of conditions and treatments that often collide with gastroparesis, and my hope is that those included in this book will be helpful to the vast majority of readers. There will always be additional conditions and questions that arise which I was not able to cover within these pages. However, the principles and concepts dis-cussed throughout the book can still be applied to an array of medical issues and concerns.

It is important to remember that gastroparesis is a chronic condition with no known cure. Although some people do have their symptoms and delayed emptying resolve over time (quite exciting!), most of us will be in it for the long haul. With this in mind, we will be placing more focus on the long-term perspective for many of our treatment discussions. For the same reason, general lifestyle considerations and the key concepts of self-advocacy will be the topics that wrap up this book.

Medications to Treat Delayed Emptying

12

A variety of medications are used in the treatment of gastroparesis. The overwhelming majority of these medications are meant to treat the symptoms that are so often associated with the condition.

Your doctor may tell you that there are medications out there for the purposes of treating gastroparesis. In this case, he is referring to a handful of medications that can simulate some form of peristalsis in the GI tract. These medications are called prokinetics because they encourage movement. Each of these medications works in very different ways and can lead to a range of effects. While you may already know that many people do not have successful responses to these drugs, some do obtain great benefit. Thus, it is important to try at least 1–2 of these options upon diagnosis.

ERYTHROMYCIN (ERYTHROCIN)

Erythromycin is actually an old antibiotic that is now rarely used in the treatment of infections. However, while it was still being prescribed for infections, it was found to stimulate the motilin receptors in the stomach. This leads to the movement of the stomach wall, which can mimic the peristalsis in this part of the GI tract that is so crucial to mechanical digestion (see page 29).

What does it do?
Causes the stomach to contract

How often do I take it?
Before every meal

How soon will it start to work?
Within the first week

What are the most common side effects?
Stomach cramping, nausea, vomiting, diarrhea

Are there drug interactions?
Multiple; consult a pharmacist

How does it come?
Tablet and liquid

Is it safe in pregnancy? Yes

Is it safe in breastfeeding? No

Special Concerns:
The benefit may lessen with time

The activity of erythromycin does not last very long. So when used for inducing stomach movements in gastroparesis, it must be taken prior to every meal. This allows it to stimulate that muscle wall while the food is in the stomach. Some people experience great success with the use of this medication, and find that it improves symptoms related to food accumulating in the stomach, such as fullness and nausea. Some will find that the initial benefit wears off over time with extended use and others will experience no improvement at all. Fortunately, you should know if this medication is working for you within the first week of taking it.

An unfortunate side effect with erythromycin is related to the reason that we are using it in the first place – stomach contractions. These can be painful and interpreted more as severe stomach cramping, which can obviously be a limitation on continued use. Additional side effects may include nausea, vomiting, and diarrhea. It's also important to be aware that a number of drug interactions exist with this medication, so if you are taking anything else, you must speak with your pharmacist about any possible issues.

This medication is available in both a tablet and liquid formulation. I will say that in comparison to many other products out there, this liquid doesn't taste all that bad! Erythromycin is safe to use in pregnancy, but should not be used while breastfeeding. Its use in breastfeeding has resulted in babies developing issues in processing their food.

METOCLOPRAMIDE (REGLAN)

Metoclopramide is also an older medication, and it actually has a wide array of uses. It works by binding to dopamine receptors throughout the body. When it binds to these receptors in the GI tract, it participates in regulating the motility of both the stomach and the intestine. It is a popular choice for use in a hospital when someone is experiencing a temporary delay in stomach emptying, such as immediately after pregnancy and delivery. It was also popular for the short-term treatment of nausea before some of our newer anti-nausea medications became available (more on those soon).

Some people with gastroparesis experience great benefit from metoclopramide, and studies have shown that it actually seems to be most beneficial to those with diabetic gastroparesis . Interestingly, this same group of people is also less likely to experience some of the side effects that come with the use of this medication. That is a great combination for those with diabetic gastroparesis to consider. Similar to erythromycin, metoclopramide's activity does not last very long and it must be taken before every meal. Fortunately, this is another medication for which you will know if it is working within the first week of taking it. At that time, your doctor may want to increase your dose, and any dose increases should start working within a week as well.

Because metoclopramide acts on the dopamine receptors, it can also cause a number of side effects. These include strange issues like tremors, major spasms, and restlessness. There is a very severe side effect that has also been associated with this medication called tardive dyskinesia. This condition results in involuntary movement of the face, neck, and arm muscles. Once this side effect develops, it never goes away. It is typically only seen when using the medication for more than 3 months, which means that every person that uses metoclopramide must make a personal decision regarding the risks and benefits of continued use at this time point.

Metoclopramide comes in a tablet and a liquid, although the liquid in this case is not quite as palatable. There is not an extensive amount of information available regarding the use of metoclopramide in pregnancy, and much of what is out there only evaluated use for 7-day stretches. While it was considered safe in those cases, this is

METOCLOPRAMIDE SNAPSHOT

What does it do?
Modulates contractions in the stomach and intestine

How often do I take it?
Before every meal

How soon will it start to work?
Within the first week

What are the most common side effects?
Tremors, spasms, restlessness

Are there drug interactions?
Very few

How does it come?
Tablet and liquid

Is it safe in pregnancy?
Most likely, but should only be used if providing great benefit

Is it safe in breastfeeding?
Most likely, but should only be used if providing great benefit

Special Concerns:
A serious, long-term side effect called tardive dyskinesia

very different than the extended use that would be required for gastroparesis. The decision to use this drug during pregnancy should only be made for women that experience an enormous symptomatic improvement with use. This medication also passes into breastmilk in small amounts. While this is likely to be safe, there is a small risk of side effects in infants, so it would, again, only be wise to continue use if it is providing great benefit for your symptoms.

DOMPERIDONE (MOTILIUM)

Domperidone is similar to metoclopramide because it works by binding to the dopamine receptors in the body. However, there is an important difference between these two drugs – domperidone does not enter the nervous system, which prevents it from causing many of those side effects that are possible with metoclopramide, including tardive dyskinesia.

For those of you that have already done some digging into your options for treatment, you might be aware that this drug isn't available in the United States. This is one of the biggest sources of confusion with this medication and has sparked a lot of theories that have been passed around. The truth is that domperidone has never been available or approved in the US. It is approved in many other countries (including Canada and across Europe) for use in GI motility disorders such as gastroparesis. It is important to clarify that it has never been denied approval in the US, either.

Domperidone is approved in many countries outside of the US for motility disorders. It does not have US approval simply because no one has done the studies necessary to obtain it.

Altogether, this means that domperidone has simply never been evaluated for approval in the United States because no company has submitted the necessary applications, documents, and trials to obtain that approval. It is not because it was pulled from the market or rejected due to safety concerns, which is a common misunderstanding.

While not available in the United States from a pharmacy, it is not impossible for someone in the US to obtain the medication. In fact, many with gastroparesis have found that they can get it from compounding pharmacies with a valid prescription. In 2007, the FDA released a statement that the compounding of domperidone is not permitted in US compounding pharmacies. Despite this, some compounding pharmacies are still filling prescriptions, although it may be difficult to find one that is willing to do this since it is not technically permitted. A limited number of doctors participate in a special access program through the FDA that provides the medication to a small number of qualified people. And finally, Canadian pharmacies will fill prescriptions from US doctors, but speak with your doctor to ensure that the pharmacy that you use to fill the prescription is reputable and legal.

Because this medication is not approved in the US and did not undergo the studies and approval process required by the FDA (see page 109), we do not have as much information on how well it works and what side effects it might cause. Based on the studies that we do have available, it appears to work well for some people with gastroparesis, including those that did not improve with metoclopramide and erythromycin. According to these studies, it also appears to be relatively safe, even with extended use. The most common side effects are dry mouth and headaches. But as I mentioned, there is limited information for this medication in comparison to what we have for other drugs.

You may be aware of the health advisories that were released in Canada regarding the risk of cardiac side effects with domperidone. The specific cardiac side effect in this case is called QT Prolongation. The term "QT" refers to a part of the electrical cycle of the heart. Certain drugs have the potential to extend this cycle. Small changes do not seem to matter, but when it is extended far enough, it can cause cardiac arrest. This is extremely rare, and usually requires a person to also have an underlying heart condition and/or to be using multiple

DOMPERIDONE SNAPSHOT

What does it do?
Modulates contractions in the stomach and intestine

How often do I take it?
Before every meal

How soon will it start to work?
Within the first week

What are the most common side effects?
Dry mouth, headache

Are there drug interactions?
Very few but some can be serious, so it is important to consult with a pharmacist

How does it come?
Powder (can place into capsules)

Is it safe in pregnancy?
Most likely, but should only be used if providing great benefit

Is it safe in breastfeeding?
Most likely, but should only be used if providing great benefit

Special Concerns:
Not available in the United States

other medications that can also cause this prolongation. In this case, the risk also increases with higher doses of domperidone.

If you have an underlying heart condition or are also using medications that can cause QT prolongation, you may be at increased risk. It would be a good idea to speak with your doctor about your risks before starting domperidone so that he can monitor your heart's activity through an EKG (electrocardiogram). Domperidone does also have some drug interactions, which can slightly increase the cardiac risk as well, so it is important to speak with your doctor or pharmacist about your other medications. But I would like to reiterate here that this side effect is extremely rare for the typical person, and your doctor is able to conduct EKGs to monitor your heart and detect any changes early on.

Much like metoclopramide, this medication also only acts for a short time and so it should be taken before meals to have an adequate effect. Higher doses of this drug may be more effective than lower doses, so dose increases may be warranted if it does not start working right away. However, it should be clear if it is helping within a week of starting and within a week of any dose change.

This medication comes in a powder that can be placed into capsules by a compounding pharmacy. There is little information available regarding the use of this medication in pregnancy, although in very small studies it appears to be safe. Due to the limited information, a mother should only continue to use this medication during pregnancy if it is greatly improving her symptoms. Similarly, small studies show that a little bit of domperidone is transferred in breastmilk but appears to be safe. Again, because these studies are small, it should only be used while breastfeeding if there is a real benefit to the mother.

Some of the medications more commonly used in those with gastroparesis that cause QT prolongation when combined with other drugs include (but are not limited to):

- Erythromycin
- Promethazine
- Ondansetron
- Granisetron

CISAPRIDE (PROPULSID)

Cisapride is similar to domperidone in many ways. However, instead of working on the dopamine receptors in the GI tract, it actually works on the serotonin receptors. It appears to be beneficial for some people with gastroparesis that have not succeeded with other medications and must be taken before every meal. It even carries the same cardiac risk of QT prolongation that is seen with domperidone.

To add yet another similarity, it is not available from pharmacies in the United States. But the story with this medication is different, because it was approved and available in the US from July 1993 until May 2000. This medication was actually withdrawn from the market due to concern for serious cardiac side effects. In fact, by the time that it was pulled, the FDA had received 341 reports of heart rhythm abnormalities and 80 deaths. In addition to causing that same QT prolongation as domperidone, cisapride can also cause other heart rhythm changes.

It appears that many of the people that experienced these side effects with cisapride fell into those higher risk groups that we talked about before – they had underlying heart conditions and/or were also using other medications that increased their risk of this effect. It is quite likely that these dangerous cardiac side effects would have been reduced if doctors had been more careful about who they were prescribing the medication for. In fact, the medical community has gained a much better understanding for handling these types of cardiac side effects since the time that this medication was removed from the market.

Regardless, cisapride is now only available through a special access program specifically for people that have not responded to other medications. This means that it is rarely used and difficult to obtain, and is only permitted for those that have severe symptoms and have failed on all

CISAPRIDE SNAPSHOT

What does it do?
Modulates contractions in the stomach and intestine

How often do I take it?
Before every meal

How soon will it start to work?
Within the first week

Special Concerns:
This medication is tightly regulated through a special access program, and all drug interactions and special situations for use, such as pregnancy, are closely defined and monitored through this program.

QT prolongation is much better understood now than it was 15 years ago. We now know when it is most likely to happen, how to reduce the risk, and how to monitor for it.

One of the reasons that we are better at managing it is because the FDA now requires that all medications be tested for this risk prior to approval. Another example of the field of medicine learning with time!

of the medications that we have already discussed. Through this special access program, there are strong safeguards placed on who can and cannot use it and what medications can be taken with it to help to prevent those cardiac side effects. Use during pregnancy and breastfeeding would also be strongly regulated within this program.

Considering the strict governmental controls on its use, I won't go into any further explanation about how and when to use the medication. But I do think it is important to understand what this medication is and why it is so difficult to obtain. Again, rumors abound regarding its safety, so it is important to set the record straight.

OTHER TREATMENTS FOR GASTROPARESIS

This short list of medications is all that we currently have available to us for simulating peristalsis in the GI tract. There are many studies being conducted on new, promising drugs for this purpose. However, I won't discuss those here because that is an area of medicine that is constantly changing, and will almost certainly be different as soon as this book is published! In fact, one of the most promising molecules out there, a ghrelin agonist called TZP-102, ended up failing in Phase 3 trials, so it is best not to get our hopes up until the research is complete (see page 109).

There are also some non-medication options for the treatment of gastroparesis, and we will take a look at those now.

Non-Medication Treatments for Delayed Emptying

13

As we saw in the previous chapter, there are not very many medications available that can help to improve the inhibited motility that causes gastroparesis. In this section, we will briefly cover the small number of non-medication treatments that are also available. Once we are done with this chapter, we will dive into the medications that are used to treat the symptoms of gastroparesis, a much more pertinent topic for the majority of us!

BOTULINUM TOXIN INJECTION (BOTOX)

Most people are familiar with the use of the Botox injection as a cosmetic treatment to slow the visible process of aging. Believe it or not, this same injection is also used for a variety of legitimate medical conditions. Each of these uses is based on the same premise – injection of Botox into the muscle can reduce muscle activity and also limit any abnormal muscle contractions that have been occurring. Its use has been evaluated in muscles throughout the body, from the head, neck, and eye, to the gastrointestinal tract.

When used for gastroparesis, Botox is injected into the pyloric sphincter with the goal of loosening the sphincter. This is thought to possibly be more effective in patients with a sphincter that may be particularly tight. The initial results with

The full name for the product that makes up Botox is a long one - onabotulinumtoxinA.

It is actually a dangerous toxin produced by a certain bacteria. It was isolated and studied and can now be used to treat a variety of conditions.

the use of this treatment were very promising – in a study of 63 people, 43% felt that their symptoms improved for up to 5 months. Based on these results alone, it suddenly became an option that GI physicians all over the country were considering for their patients.

But then someone conducted a study that compared the treatment to a placebo. And then someone else conducted another study that compared the treatment to a placebo. And the results from these two studies matched. There was no difference in the outcomes for the people that received Botox and the people that received the placebo. There appears to be a phenomenal placebo response with this treatment option that leads to a temporary improvement in some people (see page 123). But that response is purely placebo induced and does not last beyond the first 3–5 months after treatment.

In case you were wondering, the placebo in this case was a 'sham procedure' in which the patient received an endoscopy, but no injection.

This is a perfect example of the need for our gold standard studies, the RCTs (see page 20). This treatment requires endoscopy, an invasive procedure that is performed under anesthesia. During the procedure, an injection of a medication with possible side effects is made into the muscle. Because Botox only works for around 4–8 weeks, the procedure would need to be completed every couple of months, indefinitely. These conditions make this an expensive and inconvenient treatment option for those that receive it. And if we did not have placebo-controlled RCTs evaluating its efficacy, we wouldn't know that it is completely unnecessary.

UNSUPPORTED (#5)

There is a chance that some people with gastroparesis may have abnormal contractions of the pyloric sphincter (pylorospasm). If this spasm were present, it is possible that Botox may provide a true benefit in these specific cases. However, this is a very unusual finding and would not be the case for the vast majority of those with gastroparesis. Based on the available information , the 2013 guidelines for the treatment of gastroparesis included this statement, "Thus, botulinum toxin injection into the pylorus is not recommended as a treatment for gastroparesis, although there is a need for further study in patients with documented "pylorospasm".

GASTRIC ELECTRICAL STIMULATION (ENTERRA NEUROSTIMULATOR)

One of the most discussed treatment options for gastroparesis is the implantable device that can help to stimulate the stomach. This device is very different than the heart pacemakers that we are familiar with and that have been around for quite some time. The neurostimulator delivers electricity (high frequency, low energy) to the stomach in an effort to stimulate the stomach muscles to contract. It has been available in the United States under a special category of approval since 2000 and much has been learned about it since that time.

Numerous studies have been conducted that have shown that the stimulator appears to improve symptom control and quality of life, as well as tolerance for oral consumption of food. Meta-analyses have been conducted on the many available studies to draw this conclusion, and these same analyses have also found that people with diabetic gastroparesis seemed to experience the most benefit from the placement of the neurostimulator.

Studies seem to show that the stimulator is particularly beneficial for those that have diabetes-associated gastroparesis, as well as those that have come to require tube feedings.

This information means that the device may be an appropriate option for people that continue to have severe symptoms despite trying all medication therapies and lifestyle changes. This is also a great potential option for people that have come to require post-pyloric tubes for feeding, as placement of the stimulator appears to be helpful in allowing for removal of tubes and the return of oral consumption of foods (see page 155). Additionally, those with severe diabetic gastroparesis may experience a particular benefit from this device.

It is important to recognize that the decision to have this device placed should not be taken lightly.

You can read more about my experience with recovery in the Personal Experience portions of this book. Each recovery process is unique, but I have been told by a number of physicians that my experience seems to be "quite typical".

The recovery from placement is no small matter, and the devices must be replaced every 5–10 years as the battery dies. Data on the stimulators that have been placed show that movement of the leads or the development of infection around the device has occurred in up to 10% of people that have it. This is a large number of potentially very serious risks. This device is also made of metal, which means that special precautions must be taken in a number of situations and a Medical Alert should be carried at all times.

SUPPORTED (#2)

It is clear from the studies that have been conducted with the neurostimulator that it is not curative. Its usefulness lies in its ability to limit symptoms and help people in making their situations more manageable through lifestyle and dietary modifications. The decision to have the neurostimulator placed should be undertaken by you, your doctor, and your surgeon only after you have come to terms with what this device can actually offer you and have failed genuine efforts to improve your condition. As you continue to read this book, you will find more guidance and information on ways to manage the symptoms that are associated with gastroparesis. As you gain a better understanding for your condition and your options, you may find that you have the ability to bring your symptoms to a tolerable level on your own.

SURGICAL MODIFICATIONS

A number of surgical options have been considered in the treatment of extremely severe gastroparesis. These include a surgical restructuring of the pyloric sphincter (pyloroplasty), partial or whole removal of the stomach (gastrectomy), and a rerouting of the intestinal tract so that the stomach is actually connected directly to the jejunum (gastrojejunostomy). There is very limited information available on the appropriateness and effectiveness of these options.

The extreme nature of these interventions dictates that they should not be considered in any but the most severe of cases. Outside of simply making everyone aware that these options exist, I will not discuss them further. Any consideration of these surgical modifications will involve numerous comprehensive discussions with a doctor and will only be undertaken after failure of all other options.

Acid Reflux

14

I feel like I've been hinting at the acid reflux treatment section quite a bit throughout the book, so I will now give it its deserved time in the spotlight! We have already established the definition and symptoms of GERD and the fact that many people with and without gastroparesis do have this condition (see page 89). In addition to the typical experience of GERD, some of us with gastroparesis also have the experience of food coming back up into the mouth through vomiting and/or regurgitation. When the food that is vomited or regurgitated is acidic, it can cause significant discomfort in the same way that is experienced with acid reflux. This symptom also carries additional concerns, including damage to the mouth and teeth. For the purposes of this section, we will refer to any experience of acid moving into the esophagus or mouth as simply "acid reflux".

REFLUX VS. ACID REFLUX

Acid reflux: The movement of acid back into the esophagus or mouth. Acid reducers should be used to treat this.

Simple reflux: The movement of non-acidic stomach contents into the esophagus or mouth. There is no medication to treat this.

That leads me into what I believe is an incredibly important distinction that must be made and is very often ignored. There is a difference between simple reflux and acid reflux. As we just established, acid reflux involves the movement of acid back into the esophagus and, for some, into the mouth. Reflux, on the other hand, involves the movement of non-acidic stomach contents into the esophagus or mouth. Now there may be some of you for which any food that is brought up is acidic. And for those of you with feeding tubes, stomach acid can reflux quite often (see page 160). But there may be some of you who, like me, bring up a lot of food that is not acidic at all.

This is an important distinction to make because reflux that is not acidic does not need to be treated with acid reducers. Doctors often jump to prescribing medications that reduce stomach acid for anyone with gastroparesis and any type of movement of stomach contents in the wrong direction. Unfortunately, this is not always an appropriate step. In fact, acid reducers are some of the most overprescribed medications in the world.

Stomach acid serves a very important role in the digestion of the food that we eat. It is a crucial component in chemical digestion, which is made even more important in the context of gastroparesis, when our mechanical digestion is severely lacking. Using an acid reducer when it is not needed may actually inhibit our digestion and emptying times further. Stomach acid is also very important in maintaining the bacterial balance within our GI tracts by killing off many of the bacteria that we consume. Another interesting finding has been that people with low levels of acid in the stomach can experience more indigestion while eating. Using an acid reducer when it is not actually needed could cause this to happen. As you can see, it is not always appropriate to throw an acid reducer at any problem that has been labeled as 'reflux'.

Acid reducers are sometimes thought of as medications that treat reflux. The truth is, when there is no acid in that reflux, they don't do any good! And they may actually cause issues where there weren't any.

STOMACH ACID VS. FOOD ACID

There is also a distinct difference between the types of acid that can cause acid reflux. Most chronic cases of acid reflux are caused by the stomach acid that is produced by our bodies. However, acid can also be produced by some of the foods that you have eaten. This is similar to the distinction between indigestion and GERD (see page 89). If a specific food item is not being tolerated well, it may become very acidic in the stomach, and that acid may be pushed back up into the mouth or esophagus. This is an even more common occurrence for those with delayed emptying because food remains in the stomach for extended periods of time and begins to ferment and break down. This is likely the source of acid for people that only have acid reflux occur every now and then.

Identifying which of these is happening in your situation is important because it means that the medications you should be using to counteract it are different. Medications that are typically prescribed by the doctor and referred to as acid reducers will actually shut off the secretion of acid into the stomach by the body. This will have no impact whatsoever on the acid produced by a food that you have eaten.

Let's start by talking about which drugs are available to reduce acid, and then we can talk about when each medication should or should not be used.

PROTON PUMP INHIBITORS (PPIS)

PANTOPRAZOLE (PROTONIX), OMEPRAZOLE (PRILOSEC), LANSOPRAZOLE (PREVACID), RABEPRAZOLE (ACIPHEX), ESOMEPRAZOLE (NEXIUM)

PPIs are some of the most overprescribed drugs in the world, and their use has expanded even further in recent years now that many are also available over the counter (OTC). A large number of the people that currently take PPIs do not need to be on them, and long-term PPI use may not be as safe as was initially thought when they were first developed.

These medications work by blocking the proton pumps that are basically responsible for spitting hydrochloric acid into the stomach. These drugs are very effective at what they do and lead to a huge reduction in stomach acid. They also maintain this effect for a long time. If you take the pill in the morning, it will block those proton pumps for the entire day. And, on that note, you should take the pill in the morning, at least 30 minutes before breakfast.

When PPIs were first being studied, the trials did not last longer than a couple of months. But now that they are readily available and widely used, people are remaining on these medications for years. We are now learning that long-term use of these medications can increase a person's risk for some different complications, including bone fracture. It also appears that PPIs may cause absorption issues, and the people that use them for extended periods of time can become deficient in vitamin B12 and magnesium. Another increased risk is for infection, specifically pneumonia and colitis, because the stomach acid is such an important barrier in eliminating unwanted bacteria. None of these are reasons not to take the medications if you need them, but they are definitely reasons to pause and reconsider if an acid reducer is truly necessary in your situation.

The most common short term side effects that have been seen with these medications are headache, dizziness, nausea, and diarrhea. Most PPIs are supplied as a tablet or capsule, but some can also be obtained in a powder form that can be mixed with water to make a liquid (be forewarned that these taste terrible!). Lansoprazole also comes as an orally-disintegrating tablet. Some of these drugs do interact with other medications, so you should speak with your pharmacist about anything else that you are currently taking.

PPIs are believed to be relatively safe in pregnancy, although there have not been any well-conducted studies that confirm this. Some studies have shown that there may be a small but increased risk for allergies and asthma in children that were exposed to PPIs in the womb, but these studies had flaws

PPI SNAPSHOT

What does it do?
Blocks secretion of acid into the stomach

How often do I take it?
30 minutes before breakfast

How soon will it start to work?
Within 1-2 weeks

What are the most common side effects?
Headache, dizziness, nausea, diarrhea

Are there drug interactions?
Multiple, consult a pharmacist

How does it come?
Tablet, capsule, orally-disintegrating tablet, powder for liquid

Is it safe in pregnancy?
Most likely, but should only be used if providing great benefit

Is it safe in breastfeeding? Yes

Special Concerns:
Side effects can occur from long-term use, so it should only be used if truly needed

and still need to be validated through additional research. Because our knowledge is still limited, a mother should be certain that she requires this medication for control of her symptoms before continuing it in pregnancy. PPIs are also transferred in very small amounts through breastmilk, although these small amounts should generally be safe for a baby.

The use of PPIs is not limited only to the treatment of GERD. They may sometimes be prescribed for people that have an active ulcer. Reducing the stomach acid in these situations will allow the body to heal itself. In these cases, a person will typically only take the medication for 1-2 months. This class of medications is also used in the treatment of H. Pylori (see page 38), which we will discuss in more detail in a later section.

HISTAMINE-2 RECEPTOR ANTAGONISTS (H2RAS)

RANITIDINE (ZANTAC), FAMOTIDINE (PEPCID), CIMETIDINE (TAGAMET)

H2RAs used to be the drugs of choice for acid reduction before the PPIs that we just discussed hit the market. They are still used now, just less commonly. As with PPIs, they are also available either through a prescription or over the counter. Sometimes a doctor will place you on both a PPI and an H2RA. While this may be appropriate in a small number of cases, it is often unnecessary. If you are currently taking both, it would not hurt to have a conversation with your doctor about why and whether or not it is actually needed.

This group of medications works by stopping histamine from binding to histamine-2 receptors, which lowers the release of gastric acid into the stomach. These drugs are not as effective as the PPIs, so they don't lead to the same dramatic reduction in stomach acid. They also do not work for the same length of time – they must be taken twice a day, and some people will experience acid reflux close to the time that the next dose is due.

Because these medications are not quite as great at blocking acid release, they do not have as many side effects associated with using them for the long-term. However, they have still been shown to increase the risk of respiratory infections like pneumonia. While ranitidine and famotidine have very few drug interactions to worry about, cimetidine has a large number of drug interactions, so it has largely fallen out of favor.

Side effects with H2RAs are actually relatively unusual, but they have been reported to cause some headaches, nausea, dizziness, abdominal pain, and diarrhea. These medications are available in both tablet and liquid forms. The use of H2RAs in pregnancy and during breastfeeding follows the same guidance as with PPIs.

ANTACIDS

CALCIUM CARBONATE (TUMS), ALUMINUM HYDROXIDE, MAGNESIUM HYDROXIDE (MILK OF MAGNESIA) OR SOME COMBINATION OF THESE PRODUCTS

Antacids are the acid reducers that have been around "forever" and are all available over the counter, without a prescription. What most people don't realize is that antacids are completely different than other acid reducers in the way that they work. This group of medications actually reduces acid simply by binding to the acid present in the stomach at the time that they are taken. They have no impact on the body's production of stomach acid and do not differentiate between acid from the stomach and acid produced from foods.

These medications are taken when they are needed, meaning that when you feel acid refluxing into your

What does it do?
Binds to any acid in the stomach

How often do I take it?
When you experience acid reflux

How soon will it start to work?
Immediately

What are the most common side effects?
Constipation (with calcium)
Diarrhea (with magnesium)

Are there drug interactions?
They may bind to drugs present in the stomach if not separarated by about 2 hours

How does it come?
Chewable, liquid

Is it safe in pregnancy? Yes

Is it safe in breastfeeding? Yes

Special Concerns: None

esophagus, you can pop an antacid. They work pretty much immediately, because they just need to land in the stomach and start binding away. In fact, they are supplied as chewables and liquids for that exact reason. If you are already taking a PPI or an H2RA but are still experiencing some acid reflux every now and then, you can take one of these as well to help relieve that discomfort.

The side effects of these products are mostly limited to the GI tract and can actually be tailored to counteract some of the symptoms that you might have from your gastroparesis. For instance, calcium carbonate is well known for causing constipation. Magnesium hydroxide, on the other hand, is well known for causing diarrhea. So if you are prone to constipation, your antacid of choice may well be magnesium. If you are prone to diarrhea, your antacid of choice should probably be calcium carbonate. Similarly, if you have a deficiency in either of these nutrients, that should be taken into consideration when you are selecting an antacid. Aluminum hydroxide is not used as often because it is not safe for people with certain conditions, so I would generally recommend one of the other two options.

Just as these medications bind to stomach acid, they also have the potential to bind to some other drugs. However, this is a limited interaction that only lasts while the antacid is still in your stomach. So if you separate it from your medications by about 2 hours, there should be no concern for interaction. When used in moderation, calcium carbonate and magnesium hydroxide are also safe to use in pregnancy and while breastfeeding. Just keep in mind that you should not be downing excessive quantities, for both your sake and the baby's.

ACID REDUCER OR ANTACID

So now the obvious question is "Which one do I use?". That depends on your situation. If you find that you are chronically experiencing acid reflux, then you should be on a medication that blocks the secretion of acid into the stomach (PPI or H2RA). If you find that you do not experience acid reflux on a regular basis, then you should not be taking a medication regularly.

If you have acid that comes up periodically or only at certain points in time, an antacid might be the best option for you. Whether it is the food or the stomach producing this acid, the antacid will work for either (unlike an acid reducer). It works when you need it and does not need to be taken regularly. It has limited side effects and you do not have to worry about any long-term concerns. In the same way, if you need an acid reducer because you have chronic acid reflux, you can take an antacid whenever you experience 'breakthrough' acid reflux, which is most likely being caused by acid from your food.

Some of you might already be on a PPI or H2RA and are not certain if you need it. There is no harm in going off of one of these medications to see if it is actually beneficial for you. However, a unique consideration with PPIs and H2RAs is that when you miss a dose or stop using them abruptly, you may experience rebound acid reflux. This can be very uncomfortable and also very discouraging if you were testing to see if you could stop taking your medication. This rebound should only last for a couple of days, so you will need to push through it if you want to evaluate your symptoms without the medication. A good test to evaluate your symptoms should last for at least 2 weeks. If you're not sure if there is a difference, you can always try to take the medication again for about 2 weeks and compare.

Rebound acid reflux:

Occurs when a dose of PPI or H2RA is missed or stopped. Involves an increase in acid production that lasts for 2-3 days and then returns to normal.

I know that this covered a lot of information related to acid production, but I hope that it will prove helpful in allowing you to pick through your symptoms and medications to ensure that you are taking only what you need for your best quality of life.

Constipation 15

When each of us developed gastroparesis, this led to a change both in our diets and in the way that our bodies process our foods. These changes can lead to downstream effects within the GI tract, which often manifests as a change in our stool. The nature of gastroparesis means that even though diarrhea can occur, constipation is the most common result for many of us.

Constipation may seem like just a nuisance to the typical person, but when it becomes chronic it can actually result in much larger issues. Severe constipation can cause the entire intestine to back up, which, in turn, can cause the stomach to empty at an even slower rate. It can also cause significant discomfort both at rest and when attempting to defecate. Attempts to stool can lead to anal bleeding and a lot of pain in that area. Finally, very severe constipation can actually lead to intestinal impaction, which can only be fixed by the manual removal of stool.

Since none of this sounds particularly enjoyable, I think we are all quite interested in how we can manage and prevent the constipation that can so often occur with this condition. Surprisingly, the best treatment option is not a medication or supplement. It is water.

This is such an obvious factor in the development of constipation that we often forget about it. Many of us with gastroparesis end up severely restricting our water intake, for a plethora of reasons. Some of us simply cannot tolerate it and it comes back up, some cannot handle the extra volume in the stomach, and other people may have gotten a lot of their liquids from fresh foods that they are no longer eating.

We discussed the fact that water is absorbed out of the small and large intestine along with the nutrients from our food. When the body is running low on water, more and more liquid is sucked out of the intestine and into the body, leaving the stool ever drier and harder.

There are a number of ways to try to get water back into the diet. For me, my issues are with still water. I cannot drink it or it will shoot back up my throat and into my mouth. However, I do handle carbonated beverages relatively well. In order to create a palatable water-based drink that I can tolerate, I now mix a tiny amount of juice with a glass of carbonated water, and it has worked wonders in alleviating my constipation. Other people may do better with hot or warm liquids instead of cold liquids. Sometimes incorporating liquid-filled meals into the diet may also help, such as cream or broth-based soups.

An important point to be aware of is that caffeine is actually a diuretic, which means that it causes the body to eliminate more water via urine.

This explains why coffee often makes people run to the bathroom more often. But another consideration is that getting liquid through a caffeinated beverage may not increase fluid levels as much as you might hope because of this effect.

Reintroducing fresh foods that contain liquid is also a great option. Fruits contain both water and fibers that can help to loosen the stool. For instance, the melon family is brimming with liquid and is relatively easy to digest. Overripe fruit may also be easier on the stomach because it is soft and partially broken down, providing both water and fiber. For those of us with gastroparesis, a number of fruits might become more tolerable when they are peeled, so that is an option as well.

There is no doubt that increasing the fluid intake in your diet will dramatically improve constipation issues. But there are going to be times when it is not enough. A new medication, a new health condition, a symptom flare, a temporary slip in our management plans – any of those could set our GI tracts out of whack and cause the return of some constipation. And for some people, inclusion of fluids in the diet will not be enough to combat constipation. In either of those cases, there are a number of medications that can be considered.

CONSTIPATION MEDICATIONS

As a general rule, the medications used to treat constipation remain in the GI tract. They will not be absorbed into the body or enter the blood or other organs. This is a reassuring fact because it means that you do not need to be concerned about side effects in other parts of the body. These medications stay right where you need them to be for treating your symptoms.

All of the medications that we will discuss in this section are available over-the-counter, without a prescription.

There are many types of medications that can be taken to treat or prevent constipation, and each should be used for different situations. It is also possible to over-use certain products, which should be avoided. We will cover all of that here in an effort to help you personalize your medication choices to find what will work best and be safest for you.

POLYETHYLENE GLYCOL (MIRALAX)

Miralax works by binding to water, keeping it trapped within the intestine so that it is not able to be absorbed into the body. This is probably one of the most popular medications for the prevention of constipation, and there are a few reasons for this. For one thing, it doesn't impact our ability to absorb sugars or electrolytes, which can be a problem with other constipation medications. Another reason is that we are not able to develop tolerance to it. This means that just because we use Miralax every day does not mean that we have to increase the dose over time. And finally, stopping its use or missing a dose does not cause the development of worsened constipation.

This product is a powder and is typically taken on a daily basis with the average dose of one 'capful', the equivalent to 17 grams. But for the reasons that we just discussed above, each person can actually develop a unique regimen that works best for them. Doses could be a full cap, ½ cap, or 2 caps, taken every other day, twice a day, or once a day. If you find that your stools are too loose with Miralax, you can reduce the amount you take or you can reduce how often you take it. If you find it isn't quite working, you can take more per dose or take it more often. Be aware however, that as the doses get bigger and more frequent, your chances of developing urgency and diarrhea increase. This makes logical sense, and simply reducing the dose can prevent this from happening again.

It takes about 2-3 days to see the effect of Miralax. You will not immediately notice a change after the first dose that you take, so don't worry that it isn't working yet. This also means that if you would like to change your dose, it might be best to not do so more often than every 5-7 days, so that you can carefully monitor your response. By following these guidelines, you can begin to develop a regimen that is tailored especially for you.

The largest complaint with the use of Miralax is the development of gas and bloating. This can be quite significant for some people, so it is important to monitor for this and recognize if it is coming from your gastroparesis or from the use of this medication. Other than that, however, this medication is quite safe, even with long-term use. It stays in the GI tract, so it can be used safely in pregnancy and breastfeeding.

It is important to note that while Miralax is really good at breaking up newly forming stool, it does not work as well for breaking up stool that is already present. For situations in which you have severe constipation already, you may need to also take another medication initially to clear your intestines. Miralax can act as a great option for preventing the development of constipation in the future.

POLYETHYLENE GLYCOL SNAPSHOT

What does it do?
Traps water within the intestine

How often do I take it?
Depends on your symptoms

How soon will it start to work?
Within 2-3 days

What are the most common side effects?
Gas, bloating

Are there drug interactions?
No

How does it come?
Powder (mix with any liquid)

Is it safe in pregnancy? Yes

Is it safe in breastfeeding? Yes

Special Concerns: None

SENNOSIDES (SENNA), BISACODYL (DULCOLAX)

STIMULANT LAXATIVE SNAPSHOT

What does it do?
Stimulates peristalsis in the intestine

How often do I take it?
Depends on your symptoms, but no more than once a day and 3 times per week

How soon will it start to work?
Within 6-8 hours

What are the most common side effects?
Diarrhea, urgency

Are there drug interactions?
No

How does it come?
Tablet, capsule, liquid, suppository

Is it safe in pregnancy? Yes

Is it safe in breastfeeding? Yes

Special Concerns: None

Stimulant laxatives work by, as you might have guessed, stimulating the intestine. This increases peristalsis in the lower GI tract and promotes motility. They also appear to have some impact on the retention of fluid in the intestine, increasing the amount of water that stays and softens the stool. If you have been told specifically that you have slowed motility within your lower GI tract, then these medications might be an option to consider for treating your constipation.

Stimulant laxatives, however, are considered relatively unpleasant to use by many people because they can cause significant urgency and sometimes intestinal irritation. They are more likely to result in diarrhea than the use of a gentler laxative such as Miralax. Because of this, you must maintain adequate fluid intake while using these medications and recognize that they can cause you to lose extra electrolytes (such as sodium, potassium, phosphate, and magnesium). Due to these concerns, it is generally recommended not to use these more often than three times per week, and no more than one in a day. These products are available as capsules, tablets, liquids, and suppositories.

This group of medications may be particularly useful if you are experiencing severe constipation or your doctor has told you that you are very backed up. They may be beneficial to use when you are first starting to add Miralax to your regimen to help in clearing out the intestine. However, Miralax is a better long-term option for the typical person in order to avoid those issues with electrolyte changes and diarrhea. These medications are safe to use in pregnancy and while breastfeeding as long as they are not used in excess (dehydration and changes to electrolytes are not a good idea for you or your baby!).

MAGNESIUM HYDROXIDE (MILK OF MAGNESIA)

This product is considered an osmotic laxative because it works by pulling water into the intestine from the rest of the body. This water entering the gut rapidly softens and loosens the stool. It has a much faster and stronger activity than Miralax, which can lead to more urgency and diarrhea. If it is not well tolerated or too much is taken, it may also cause cramping.

If you are using this to prevent the development of constipation, always try to start with the smallest dose. If it does not work after a few days, increase the dose slowly. This product comes as both a liquid and a chewable, and in fact, you might remember that we discussed this medication when we were talking about acid reflux. If you use this medication to treat an episode of acid reflux, it is very important to remember that you just took a laxative – it might be best not to take any additional doses that day!

Just as with stimulant laxatives, this can cause a lot of water loss. This makes sense because we know that it works by pulling water out of the body and into the intestine. Thus, it is very important to remain well-hydrated when you are using this product. There is also the potential for you to absorb additional magnesium over time with the long-term use of this medication, so if you are planning to use this for an extended period, be sure to let your doctor know so that he can evaluate your blood levels.

MAGNESIUM HYDROXIDE SNAPSHOT

What does it do?
Pulls water into the intestine

How often do I take it?
Depends on your symptoms, but no more than once a day

How soon will it start to work?
Within 8 hours

What are the most common side effects?
Diarrhea, urgency, cramping

Are there drug interactions?
No

How does it come?
Chewable, liquid

Is it safe in pregnancy? Yes

Is it safe in breastfeeding? Yes

Special Concerns: None

DOCUSATE (COLACE)

Docusate is considered a stool softener which functions by lowering the surface tension of the stool and allowing it to mix more easily with water. It does not cause any type of forceful movement like you might see with stimulant or osmotic laxatives. In fact, it is even more gentle than Miralax. This can be a good or a bad thing. For those of you that already have significant constipation, docusate will not be helpful in resolving this issue. However, it can be useful for keeping the stool in a softer state when taken every day. This may be an option for those of you that have a lot of straining, pain, or bleeding, but do not tolerate Miralax well.

This medication is taken daily and comes as a capsule or liquid. The typical adult can take anywhere from 50mg to 200mg safely every day. It will take a few days to begin to see any effect from its use. Side effects with this medication are incredibly unusual, and there are also no long-term concerns with its use. Because it stays in the GI tract, it can be used safely in pregnancy and with breastfeeding.

MAGNESIUM CITRATE

This is a very different product than the other magnesium - hydroxide - that we already discussed. It also works by drawing water into the intestine from the rest of the body. However, it does this at an accelerated rate, which causes an irritation of the intestine and rapid expulsion of its contents.

This product comes in a glass bottle as a clear, flavored liquid. It is very important to understand and recognize that the use of this product is intended to produce a sudden and significant expulsion of the contents of the gut. In the medical field it is sometimes referred to as a 'grenade in the bowels'. This is not a product that is to be used daily in the maintenance of regular stools. Its use is limited to only those situations in which the intestines need to be cleared of their contents.

The entire bottle is to be consumed at once and its effect typically occurs somewhere between 30 minutes to 6 hours after consumption. Due to the rapid results and loss of water that this product can produce, it is very important to stay well-hydrated while using it. Besides the expected urgency that it can cause, side effects also include stomach pain and nausea and vomiting. The liquid is more palatable when it has been chilled prior to use.

If you have any type of kidney dsyfunction, be cautious about using this product, as it can lead to dangerous magnesium build-up in the body. This product is safe to use in pregnancy and breastfeeding as long as it is used only in the unusual case of significant constipation.

ENEMAS

Enemas work by clearing out the stool inside of the colon. They do not cause any changes to the small intestine, but if there is a large buildup of stool in the colon, then an enema may help to open up room for movement throughout the intestine. They might be helpful in cases of severe constipation in an effort to force movement of the stool. The use of any enemas should be limited whenever possible. They are never appropriate to be used on a regular basis for the treatment of constipation. They can cause you to become dehydrated and can also lead to changes in your electrolytes that are important to the regular function of the body. Additionally, they do not help to prevent constipation, so if you have chronic issues, another treatment option will be safer and easier for you to implement. Any time that you use an enema, be sure to take in a lot of water as well to replenish what is being eliminated.

MINERAL OIL

This may be used to soften and lubricate the stool that is currently present in the rectum. If you know that you have a hard buildup of stool in that area, this may be an appropriate choice. It will typically work within 2-15 minutes, but a second dose should not be used if the first does not work.

BISACODYL

We discussed stimulant laxatives already in their other forms, but bisacodyl also comes as an enema. It is typically preferable to use the suppository instead of the enema if at all possible, as the suppository is less damaging and both will lead to an effect within 15–60 minutes. A second dose should not be used if the first does not work.

SODIUM PHOSPHATES (FLEETS)

I want to clarify that a number of enemas are sold under the brand name Fleets. However, the sodium phosphates enema is the standard product that a doctor is referring to when he uses that term. If you are unsure of which one to use, be sure to clarify, as each enema is very different. Sodium phosphates work by causing water to pour into the lower intestine and rapidly induce peristalsis. An effect should be seen within 1–3 hours of use, and a second dose should not be used if the first dose not work.

MANAGING CONSTIPATION

As you can see, there are a variety of options available in the treatment of constipation. And because all of these products are available over the counter, you are able to be in full control of your own care. That being said, it is always a great idea to run any changes or ideas by your doctor or pharmacist, as well as any specific concerns you have after trying some of your options.

There are also some prescription medications that can treat constipation. However, these drugs are meant to treat actual dysfunction of the intestines, and are not recommended for the standard case of gastroparesis.

While these medications may be necessary in some cases, they are not mentioned here for this reason, and should not be used until the other available options have been exhausted.

Again, management of constipation by increasing water and liquid intake will always be the most sustainable and manageable approach. Even at times when increased fluid intake is not adequate on its own, it is still a necessary component in the treatment of constipation.

If you need to use laxatives, then start with the gentler options first in order to avoid uncomfortable and frustrating side effects. Pay attention to your response and tweak your doses as needed to obtain the most comfort. Be careful when using any drastic measures, such as enemas, and always use these products in moderation.

Nausea

16

For many with gastroparesis, nausea is the most debilitating symptom. Most people can learn to deal with the frustrations of acid reflux, constipation, bloating, and pain. But nausea can be very hard to overcome. There are many different ways that nausea can present, and it can be anywhere from mild to severe. Some people will find that it is worst in relation to sudden movements or a type of motion sickness, others will find that it is present all of the time. It may get worse during a flare or it may be triggered by specific foods or smells.

Every person will need to pay close attention to their own situations in order to identify what worsens and improves their nausea. This will help to clarify if it is related to motion, food, smell, or fullness, etc. The management for nausea will also be different for people that experience it consistently than for people that have bouts that flare up at unexpected times. Lifestyle and habit changes are hugely important in battling nausea, and medications can be an important weapon as well.

NON-MEDICATION TREATMENTS

My personal experience with this symptom is what I refer to as "baseline nausea" – it seems to be present at all times on some level. The majority of

---

the time it presents at a low level that I have learned to live normally with, but must be careful not to throw out of whack. For instance, I have had many people comment that I move gracefully, which is really just a nice way of saying that I turn, stand, and bend very slowly. Training myself to move this way consistently has helped to prevent a lot of nauseated episodes, but it took time to engrain! Knowing that I am now prone to become nauseated with certain activities, such as reading in the car (which didn't used to be the case), allows me to avoid them whenever possible. Recognizing days on which I am already experiencing more nausea than usual, I avoid certain foods and drinks, such as alcoholic beverages.

The first step in managing your nausea is understanding your triggers. Pay attention to the wide array of potential causes, such as foods, smells, movements, situations, and more.

These are all examples of ways to accommodate a new symptom in our lives without having to rely on medications that can cause side effects. But I also experience days on which my nausea is completely out of my control and I have no choice but to take medications so that I can feel human again. Some home remedies may be helpful to try for limiting nausea without using medications. Vitamin B6 (pyridoxine) and ginger have both been shown to improve symptoms of nausea during pregnancy. There are no studies that look at whether or not they are helpful in gastroparesis. However, these are easy items to add into any diet, so it might be helpful to try to increase your intake. In fact, I find that the smell and taste of ginger has a surprising impact on my nausea. It is important to point out that taking a ginger supplement is unlikely to have the desired effect because it seems to be the pungency of ginger that leads to an improvement.

Many of the 'natural' nausea treatments that you will find on the drugstore shelf are actually homeopathic therapies (see page 131). Carefully consider our discussion about these remedies before purchasing them. You will also notice that some of the natural treatment options actually contain flavors that are soothing to certain people, such as ginger and mint. It might not be a bad idea to experiment with various flavors and scents from their original source – you can purchase ginger and mint from the produce department and lavender from the gardening department. Experimenting may allow you to see if any scents or flavors offset your nausea and allow you to find ways to incorporate them into your management plan.

Some people also find that carbonation can be leveling and soothing to the stomach, often in the form of tonic water or ginger ale. In contrast, an old home remedy for nausea is actually cola syrup and some people find it helpful to drink flat, uncarbonated soda when they are nauseated. Every situation is different!

OVER-THE-COUNTER (OTC) MEDICATIONS

These medications are available without a prescription and are typically meant for the treatment or prevention of motion sickness. Many of us are now more prone to motion sickness than we used to be, so these may be important options to manage nausea in certain situations.

DIPHENHYDRAMINE (BENADRYL)

Diphenhydramine is actually an anti-allergy medication that works by blocking the activity of histamine in our bodies. In addition to the treatment of allergies, it has also been used to treat nausea and help people to fall asleep. One of the biggest drawbacks with this medication is that the sleep component can't be shut off – if you are using it for nausea, it is still going to make you really sleepy. A person should never take this when they need to drive or perform any other high functioning tasks. Diphenhydramine can also contribute to a hangover feeling once you wake up.

This medication will start to lose its effect for sleep and nausea over time with extended use. This means that it cannot be used consistently for either of these reasons because we eventually become tolerant to it. With periodic use it can

Just as certain tastes and smells can trigger nausea, other tastes and smells can be used to alleviate it!

DIPHENHYDRAMINE SNAPSHOT

What does it do?
Blocks histamine activity

How often do I take it?
When you are nauseated; no more than every 4-6 hours

How soon will it start to work?
Within 1 hour

What are the most common side effects?
Sleepiness, blurry vision, constipation

Are there drug interactions?
Very few

How does it come?
Tablet, capsule, liquid

Is it safe in pregnancy?
Most likely, but should only be used if providing great benefit

Is it safe in breastfeeding? No

Special Concerns:
When used repeatedly, its usefulness begins to wear off

cause constipation and can make vision blurry. It is available as a tablet, capsule, or liquid and can be taken every 4-6 hours as needed. This medication is not typically recommended for use in pregnancy or with breastfeeding, so other options should be considered in these cases.

Due to the side effects and limited benefit, this is generally not a drug of choice for the treatment of gastroparesis-related nausea, but it is often used so I wanted to make sure that we covered it here.

MECLIZINE (ANTIVERT, TRAVEL SICKNESS, NON-DROWSY DRAMAMINE)

This medication is also available in prescription form at a higher strength than what you can obtain over the counter. It is very similar to diphenhydramine in the way that it acts. It also causes drowsiness and blurry vision, although it typically makes people much less sleepy than they become with diphenhydramine. Its primary use is for the treatment and prevention of motion sickness, so it should not be used for other types of nausea that you might be experiencing.

In addition to the reduction in drowsiness, this medication is also a nice improvement over diphenhydramine because it can work for an entire day. This can be taken once a day in an effort to prevent motion sickness that day. It is available only as a tablet and a chewable tablet. Information on the use of meclizine in pregnancy and with breastfeeding is limited, but it appears to be relatively safe and may be used with the advice of a physician if it is providing great benefit.

PRESCRIPTION MEDICATIONS

PROCHLORPERAZINE (COMPAZINE), PROMETHAZINE (PHENERGAN)

These medications are both part of a class called phenothiazines, which refers to the structure of

MECLIZINE SNAPSHOT

What does it do?
Blocks histamine activity

How often do I take it?
Once daily

How soon will it start to work?
Within 1-2 hours

What are the most common side effects?
Sleepiness, blurry vision, constipation

Are there drug interactions?
Very few

How does it come?
Tablet, chewable

Is it safe in pregnancy?
Most likely, but should only be used if providing great benefit

Is it safe in breastfeeding? Yes

Special Concerns:
Best used to prevent, not to treat, the nausea related to motion sickness

the drug molecule. Much like diphenhydramine and meclizine, these drugs also work by inhibiting histamine from functioning in the body. However, they are more effective at doing this in the parts of the brain that are associated with the nausea response, specifically a location called the chemo-receptor trigger zone.

As you might expect from the way that they work, both of these medications can cause significant drowsiness. This again limits their use if you need to be able to drive, go to work, or perform other activities on the day that you are taking them. They must also be taken every 6 hours, which makes them better for use with bouts of nausea as opposed to consistent nausea. These medications also cause that same blurry vision and constipation that happens with the other drugs we have already discussed, as well as some possible confusion and dizziness. An additional consideration with this class of medications is QT prolongation when combined with other drugs that have the same effect.

Phenothiazines are available as tablets and liquids. They can be used in pregnancy in moderation (lower doses, limited use) if they are providing a true benefit, but are not recommended for use while breastfeeding and other options should be considered in their place. While these medications used to serve an important purpose in the treatment of nausea, they are used less commonly now that we have another class of drugs available, which we will discuss next.

5-HT3 RECEPTOR ANTAGONISTS

ONDANSETRON (ZOFRAN), GRANISETRON (SANCUSO), DOLASETRON (ANZEMET), PALONOSETRON (ALOXI)

The term 5-HT3 refers to a very specific type of receptor in the body that binds to serotonin. This is a chemical that many of you are likely familiar with from the popular psychiatric medications that

PHENOTHIAZINE SNAPSHOT

What does it do?
Blocks histamine activity

How often do I take it?
When you are nauseated; no more than every 6 hours

How soon will it start to work?
Within 1 hour

What are the most common side effects?
Sleepiness, blurry vision, constipation, confusion

Are there drug interactions?
Very few

How does it come?
Tablet, liquid

Is it safe in pregnancy?
Likely safe with limited use of small doses; should only be used if providing great benefit

Is it safe in breastfeeding? No

Special Concerns: None

What does it do?
Blocks specific serotonin activity

How often do I take it?
When you are nauseated; no
more than every 8 hours

How soon will it start to work?
Within 30-60 minutes

**What are the most common
side effects?**
Headache, fatigue, constipation

Are there drug interactions?
Multiple; consult a pharmacist

How does it come?
Tablet, orally-disintegrating
tablet, liquid, patch

Is it safe in pregnancy?
Likely, but should only be used if
providing great benefit and other
options have been exhausted

Is it safe in breastfeeding?
Not recommended unless truly
needed

Special Concerns: None

act on it. Although serotonin has become a hot topic in psychiatry, it is actually active in many different processes throughout the body. When these medications block the 5-HT3 receptor, this occurs in both the intestine and in the brain. Preventing serotonin from binding at these sites prevents the signal that is used to relay nausea.

When these medications were first released, they were limited to use only for those experiencing nausea from chemotherapy. At that time, they were incredibly expensive, and obtaining only 6-8 pills a month was more than most people were able to afford. Since that time, ondansetron and granisetron have become very affordable options, and with that affordability, their use has expanded to a number of additional types of nausea, for which they appear to also be quite effective.

Some of the more common side effects seen with these medications are headache, fatigue, and constipation. The fatigue and constipation are much less than what occurs with use of the other medications that we have discussed thus far, making these by far the most tolerable anti-nausea medications that we have available to us. They are also very versatile – you can obtain these products in tablets, orally-disintegrating tablets, liquids, and even a patch that is worn on the skin. These extra options can be nice when you are experiencing nausea that is also causing vomiting. When more than one dose is needed, it can be taken every 8 hours, but it is not typically recommended to take them around the clock continuously.

There are some drug interactions that can occur with these medications, so it is important to speak with your pharmacist about anything else that you are taking. The safety of 5-HT3 receptor antagonists during pregnancy is still somewhat unclear, but appears to be relatively safe and and may be used when providing a great benefit and other medications have failed to work. Studies related to the use of these medications while breastfeeding are limited and these molecules are expected to be present in breastmilk, so it is recommended to avoid use whenever possible and consult with a physician.

TRIMETHOBENZAMIDE (TIGAN)

This is a much older anti-nausea medication that was originally approved to treat the nausea and vomiting associated with acute GI infections. It is not very commonly used, but some doctors will turn to it when other medications do not work, so I wanted to include some information about it here. This medication is one where we are not entirely sure how it works, but we do know that it seems to have some effect on dopamine as well as serotonin.

Side effects with this medication are not very common, unless you use it while you are dehydrated, in which case it can increase the risk of some serious nervous system side effects. It is important to make sure that you have been drinking adequate fluids when you take this, which is sometimes difficult with gastroparesis, especially when you are nauseated. Otherwise, the side effects that are typically seen are the ones that I keep repeating over and over again in this section – blurry vision and drowsiness. It is the only medication in this section that does not cause constipation, but it is important to note that the constipation with 5-HT3 Antagonists is typically mild and not a reason to avoid using them.

Trimethobenzamide is available as a capsule and a suppository (an option in situations where you are experiencing a lot of vomiting) and is taken every 6-8 hours while the nausea lasts. Its use in pregnancy is generally not recommended unless non-medication options are not working to control severe nausea and you have discussed its use with your physician. It has not been studied with breastfeeding so it is best not to use it in these situations more often than single doses taken only periodically when the nausea is difficult to tolerate.

What does it do?
Unclear; various possibilities

How often do I take it?
When you are nauseated; no more than once every 6-8 hours

How soon will it start to work?
Within 30-60 minutes

What are the most common side effects?
These are unusual; blurry vision and drowsiness

Are there drug interactions?
Very few

How does it come?
Capsule and suppository

Is it safe in pregnancy?
Not recommended unless truly needed

Is it safe in breastfeeding?
Only for limited single doses taken when needed for nausea

Special Concerns:
You must stay hydrated while taking this medication

DRONABINOL (MARINOL)

What does it do?
Acts on cannabinoid receptors

How often do I take it?
When you are nauseated; no more than every 6-8 hours

How soon will it start to work?
Within 1-2 hours

What are the most common side effects?
Appetite stimulation, abdominal pain, dizziness, mood swings, drowsiness, paranoia, dysphoria

Are there drug interactions?
Multiple; consult a pharmacist

How does it come?
Capsule

Is it safe in pregnancy? No

Is it safe in breastfeeding? No

Special Concerns:
People may develop tolerance over time; this medication shows up on drug tests

Many people are aware of this medication because it has received some controversial publicity. It is actually a chemical that is found in marijuana, but the medication version is created in the lab and is not pulled from the plant itself. The receptor that this chemical acts on is found throughout the brain, and seems to have some effect in reducing feelings of nausea, particularly in patients that are receiving chemotherapy.

There have been no studies that evaluate whether or not this medication is useful in gastroparesis or for the nausea and vomiting associated with any GI conditions. One of the reasons that it has not been considered as an ideal option for those with gastroparesis is that it stimulates appetite. In fact, it is so effective at doing this that it was actually approved by the FDA for the treatment of anorexia and other conditions in which people have reduced appetites. There have also been cases where stopping this medication has led to an increase in vomiting for some people. And finally, many who take this for a long time end up developing some tolerance to its effect.

These represent a number of reasons that dronabinol should not be considered for the typical person with gastroparesis. Some of the most common side effects with this medication are abdominal pain, dizziness, drowsiness, mood swings, paranoia, and dysphoria (a feeling of unease or dissatisfaction). A number of possible drug interactions exist with this medication as well.

Dronabinol is available only as a capsule. Use during pregnancy is not recommended as there is the potential for early birth and reduced growth, as well as possible developmental delays. Use is also not recommended during breastfeeding due to the potential for serious risks in exposed infants. Another common question regarding this medication is whether it will show up on drug tests. The answer is yes – this is a component of marijuana that these tests are designed to detect.

MANAGING NAUSEA

Truly understanding and evaluating your nausea and its triggers is key to developing a management plan that will allow you to regain your quality of life. It is crucial to learn to understand, accommodate, and prevent your nausea whenever possible through lifestyle changes and considerations. There may also be simple scent or flavor options that you can add in that may help to keep it at bay.

When these changes and interventions fall short, medications are available. You saw here that there is a standout option – the 5-HT3 antagonists – that seems to work well, has multiple formulations, and causes far fewer limiting side effects. This is a medication class that could be taken while you are at work and trying to maintain your composure without having to leave for the day. Not every person will have the desired benefit from these medications, however, so the other options that we have discussed should be reviewed and considered as well.

It is important to point out that taking multiple anti-nausea medications at once does not seem to be helpful, and is also not a good idea because so many of the side effects with these medications can pile up on top of each other. If your doctor has recommended or prescribed two different medications, these medications can be alternated instead of taken together, allowing you to leverage both medications and possibly take each of them less often. With perseverance, every person can pull together a unique combination of changes and treatments that will help them to keep their nausea in check.

ALTERNATING MEDICATIONS

If the medications that have been prescribed are to be taken every 6-8 hours, then you could take only one of the medications every 4-6 hours, switching between the products each time that a dose is needed. Taking them at the same time may lead to more side effects and less benefit. Alternating them is a possible way to reduce your total usage and increase your benefit. You can discuss your specific options with your pharmacist.

Modifying Gut Bacteria

17

We have already spent plenty of time in this book discussing the bacteria that live in our guts. We've looked at how they are dispersed throughout our intestines and many of the benefits that they provide to us. In certain cases, bacteria that are exactly where we expect them to be and working exactly as they should can cause GI symptoms in people with specific intolerances, such as carbohydrate or lactose intolerance. In other cases, normal gut bacteria can take up residence in places where they don't belong or unusual bacteria can multiply and cause disturbances in our GI function.

In this section we will take a look at the accepted and theorized treatment options for some of these situations. Some of these treatments are well established, whereas others are still being researched and tested in order to gain a clearer understanding. We will also discuss a treatment option that has become all the rage in recent years in relation to gut bacteria – probiotics.

HELICOBACTER PYLORI (H. PYLORI) TREATMENTS

We have mentioned this condition a few times in the book. H. pylori is a type of bacteria that thrives in what used to be considered an uninhabitable environment – strong acid. The discovery that a bacteria existed which could survive in the acidic environment found in our stomachs was quite shocking. I won't repeat our previous discussion on the ways that the symptoms of H. pylori infection can overlap with gastroparesis symptoms, but I will reiterate that it is a very good idea to be tested for this infection via a breath test or a stool test (see page 38).

The treatment for this condition is not quite as simple as the test, and requires the combination of three or four different medications that must be taken together for 7-14 days. It is vital that all of the drugs are used in combination, or it will greatly reduce the level of success found with the treatment.

You may also hear H. pylori treatment referred to as Triple Therapy or Quad Therapy.

It is standard for a doctor to prescribe two different antibiotics. These two different antibiotics are targeted at killing the H. pylori that has taken up residence in your stomach. The other medication that is always included in this regimen is a PPI, which we discussed in the acid reflux section (see page 180). Regardless of whether or not you experience acid reflux, it is crucial to take the PPI as part of this treatment. Using an acid reducer makes your stomach less acidic, which makes it a less desirable environment for the H. pylori that are living there. This causes the bacteria to slow their growth, making them an easier target for the antibiotics that you are taking.

All of the antibiotics that are used can typically be found in liquid forms. The PPI that is prescribed is also probably available in a powder formulation that can be mixed with water. It is important to recognize that the antibiotics will need to be taken more than once a day, so during the 1-2 weeks that you are completing this therapy, you will be required to take multiple doses of medication each day, which can become burdensome. But if you stick it out, the treatment is very effective, and can lead to a large reduction in symptoms for many people.

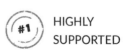 HIGHLY SUPPORTED

SMALL INTESTINAL BACTERIAL OVERGROWTH (SIBO) TREATMENTS

We have discussed the implications of SIBO in a previous section of this book (see page 94), so in this area we will limit our discussion to the possible treatments for this condition. It is important to recognize that although SIBO is an established and diagnosable medical condition, we are still learning about the best ways to treat it. Research is still underway in this area and a variety of ideas exist regarding the optimal way to keep it under control.

PREVENTION

First, let's discuss prevention. The use of an acid reducer increases a person's chances of developing SIBO. This occurs because acid reducers prevent the acid that would normally be present in your stomach from killing off some of the bacteria that you eat. This allows bacteria found in the foods that you consume to possibly survive and migrate into either your small or large intestine. It is important to confirm whether or not you truly need an acid reducer, and also to confirm that you are using the right one at the right dose. For instance, we have already discussed the fact that PPIs are much more effective at reducing stomach acid than H2RAs, so you can imagine which class is more likely to increase the risk of SIBO (see page 180).

Another consideration for preventing SIBO is to limit your use of medications that can slow the motility in the intestine. Some people with gastroparesis actually have normal motility in their intestines, while others do experience delays. Regardless of your current state, certain medications can further slow this motility, which gives bacteria an increased opportunity to move in the wrong direction. We have already mentioned some of these medications, with opioids and tricyclic antidepressants being some of the biggest offenders (see page 60). While there are definitely situations in which these medications are appropriate to use, it is important to make sure that they are necessary considering this additional risk.

ANTIBIOTICS

Antibiotics are the undisputed treatment of choice for diagnosed SIBO, but we are still working out exactly which antibiotics are best and how long they should be used for. It is important to clarify that even when these medications have been shown to lead to improvements, they do not appear to completely eliminate symptoms or 'cure' the condition.

While a large variety of antibiotics have been studied for this condition, there are two medications that have stood out thus far both for their safety and efficacy. These two antibiotics are rifaximin (Xifaxin) and neomycin (Neocin). These medications are not absorbed into the blood stream. This means that they stay within the GI tract and will not cause side effects in any other parts of the body. These are also the antibiotics that have most consistently been shown to work in treating SIBO, even in placebo-controlled trials. In addition to working, these drugs have been better tolerated than many of the other antibiotics that have been tested, which is likely related to the fact that they stay within the GI tract.

When these medications are used for the treatment of SIBO, they are typically taken 2-3 times a day for 2 weeks. Most bacteria can be treated with only one of these antibiotics. For some situations in which very specific bacterial species are present, these two antibiotics are more effective when used in combination. So while they should be used separately for the majority of cases, there are times when using them together is appropriate. It is possible that some people will have SIBO and its symptoms return even after experiencing a benefit from one of these medications, so these antibiotics have also been studied to see if they are effective a second time around. In most cases, they do appear to have a positive effect.

RIFAXIMIN SNAPSHOT

What does it do?
Kills bacteria in the gut

How often do I take it?
Three times a day

How soon will it start to work?
Within 1-2 weeks

What are the most common side effects?
Dizziness, fatigue, headache, nausea

Are there drug interactions?
Multiple; consult a pharmacist

How does it come?
Tablet

Is it safe in pregnancy? Yes

Is it safe in breastfeeding? Yes

Special Concerns: None

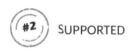 SUPPORTED

NEOMYCIN SNAPSHOT

What does it do?
Kills bacteria in the gut

How often do I take it?
Two times a day

How soon will it start to work?
Within 1-2 weeks

What are the most common side effects?
Nausea, vomiting, diarrhea, skin rash, irritation

Are there drug interactions?
Very few

How does it come?
Tablet, liquid

Is it safe in pregnancy? No

Is it safe in breastfeeding? Yes

Special Concerns:
Although it is poorly absorbed, long-term use of neomycin can cause hearing issues.

Both of these antibiotics are available as tablets, and neomycin is also available as a liquid. There are some drug interactions with these medications, so you should speak with a pharmacist about anything else that you are taking. Neomycin crosses the placenta and is not considered safe in pregnancy. Rifaximin, on the other hand, is considered to be likely safe for use in pregnancy. Because they stay within the GI tract, both of these antibiotics are considered likely safe for use during breastfeeding.

 UNSUPPORTED

Some other antibiotics have also been utilized in "drug cocktails" to treat SIBO. However, the use of a barrage of antibiotics at one time has not been shown to lead to more improvement. Instead, this actually causes a lot of side effects, and any unnecessary use of antibiotics increases the risk for the bacteria in your GI tract to develop resistance. If your doctor suggests a treatment that uses a large number of medications at once, it would be a good idea to have a discussion about whether you can try a simpler regimen first, possibly with one of the two antibiotics that we already discussed.

PROBIOTICS

Probiotics have become quite a popular topic recently. If you watch TV, they seem to be able to cure everything that is GI-related! I bet you can guess what I'm going to say next – probiotics are alternative therapies. To be more specific, they are classified as either dietary supplements or medical foods. This means that they carry the risks related to poor quality and poor manufacturing practices.

But first, let's define what these products actually are. It turns out that there are a lot of other terms that should be clarified in order to fully understand the most popular term – probiotic. Each one is important to understanding why these products have become so prevalent and are claimed to do so many things.

- **Prebiotic:** A substance that encourages the growth of certain types of bacteria. This includes the oligosaccharides found in human milk.

- **Probiotic:** A bacteria that is naturally found in the gut, and can also be placed there by taking a supplemental probiotic product

- **Postbiotic:** A byproduct of the bacteria in the gut that influences our bodies. This includes fatty acids that help build our immune systems.

- **Synbiotic:** Products that contain both probiotics and prebiotics

- **Functional Foods:** Foods that are modified to contain a prebiotic, probiotic, or postbiotic

OK! That was a lot, but hopefully now the term "probiotic" actually makes more sense. And it also makes sense why these products have received so much attention. If many of the issues in our GI tract relate to disturbances in our gut flora, then the logical correction for this would be to add the good flora back into our guts. Right?

Unfortunately, it's not that easy. There are many (and when I say many, I almost mean endless) different types of probiotics on the market. Each bottle that you pick up will have a slightly different type of bacteria or bacterial strain, and each bottle will probably also contain a different quantity of that bacteria. Although an enormous number of studies have been completed that look at the usefulness of probiotics in treating a variety of GI conditions, the types and numbers of bacteria used in these studies are all different. In fact, many of these studies use strains that aren't even available to purchase. To make it even worse, when these studies are looked at as a whole in meta-analyses, probiotics don't seem to work very well.

The science of probiotics is very young, but the media, supplement, and food industries have

You have probably seen many of these differences when you were perusing the drugstore shelves, like this shower of names:

lactobacillus, bifidobacterium, saccharomyces, acidophilus

And the quantities of these different species can range by 100,000-fold.

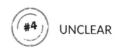 **#4** UNCLEAR

exploded it into the mainstream long before it was ready. You will now find functional foods all over the place that are 'full of probiotics'. There are a wide array of products on the shelf that claim to improve digestion through pre-, pro-, and post-biotics, even though they have not actually been shown to do this. And for how prevalent these products are, this industry is fully unregulated, so it is often difficult to know that what you are buying is what you are actually getting (unless, of course, you find a third-party certified product (see page 119)).

BENEFITS

I've already mentioned that the studies conducted on probiotics have been disappointing. Because they use so many different strains and quantities of bacteria, the findings for many of these small studies have not been duplicated. And in cases where similar studies were conducted, the outcomes did not agree with each other. This leaves us very confused about whether or not probiotics actually have a place for treatment in many conditions. We do, however, know that two specific probiotics appear to be useful in very targeted situations.

I would like to clarify again that I have no conflicts of interest and have no relationship with the companies that make these products.

In a previous position that I held, I conducted an exhaustive review of probiotics and contacted a large number of companies to evaluate their product quality. These two were the clear winners.

PROMISING

1. I had mentioned before that when we take antibiotics, they have the potential to cause diarrhea when they kill off some of the normal bacteria that are found in our intestines (see page 39). It makes sense that in order to prevent this side effect, we would want to see if we can simply supplement those bacteria that are being killed. Surprisingly, however, most studies with different types of bacteria have not actually been successful in doing this. Lactobacillus rhamnosus (Culturelle) is the exception, as it appears to help decrease the diarrhea seen with antibiotics in both children and adults, although the evidence is not very strong. Although Culturelle is not third-party certified, the company that makes this product was willing to provide me with information regarding its quality. The

biggest drawback with this product is the high cost, so seriously consider how important it is to possibly prevent diarrhea before purchasing this product.

2. VSL#3 appears to be effective in treating IBS, ulcerative colitis, and pouchitis. In fact, the studies conducted with this probiotic are some of the best ones out there, and it has been shown consistently to lead to improvement in these severe GI conditions. This is another company that was able to provide me with proof of quality when I contacted them. However, it is an incredibly expensive product and the known benefits appear to be limited to these specific GI conditions. Its use is not generally recommended for any other reasons and it has not been studied in gastroparesis.

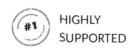 HIGHLY SUPPORTED

RISKS

Although we have very little information on the benefits that probiotics might bring, we do actually have a good deal of information on some of the risks that come with them. In order to really understand these risks, we need to have a better understanding for what these products actually are – capsules or packets full of living, breathing bacteria. This is quite different than anything else that we have discussed thus far, be it medications, supplements, or foods.

Bacteria are living organisms!

When you look at the Supplement Facts for a probiotic product, it usually states the number of bacteria in a capsule or packet. This quantity is described in CFU, which stands for colony forming units, and basically means a single bacterium. Culturelle, for instance, states that it contains 2.5 billion CFU, which means that it contains 2.5 billion bacteria. That is a lot! And yet, when I called these companies to look into their product quality, they sent me information showing that the capsules actually contained 25 billion bacteria. That is 10 times more! When I asked the company why the information they sent showed a ten-fold

Here we go with the numbers again!

2.5 billion ≈ 2,500,000,000

difference than what was listed on the box, they stated that extra bacteria are added to the product so that as they die off, there will still be more than 2.5 billion in there when the product reaches its expiration date.

That was surprising information to me, and yet it was confirmed by many other probiotic manufacturers. It is definitely not reassuring to hear that there may be 10x the number of bacteria in the product than what I am expecting. But there is also another concern present with a product made of bacteria – contamination. It is incredibly common for labs to experience contamination when they are working with bacteria. Bacterial contamination could be a very similar strain, or it could be a much different and dangerous strain that can cause severe infections. This type of contamination has occurred before in poor quality probiotics and will occur again. Thus, quality is of particular importance with these products.

Finally, the last point that I want to make regarding possible risks with probiotics is in relation to what happens when they end up in places other than the GI tract. There have been many reports of severe infections that have caused hospitalization and death because probiotics were used when they should not have been.

HARMFUL #6

If any of the following situations applies to you, probiotic use should be avoided:

1. **Dental Surgery**

   If you are going to have dental surgery, take a couple days off of your probiotics. You don't want to risk the bacteria entering your blood stream from your mouth.

2. **Drugs that Suppress the Immune System**

   If you are taking a medication that suppresses your immune system, you are at increased risk for infection. In fact, there have been many reports of people on immunosuppressant medications that have developed severe bloodstream infections from probiotics. If you are not sure which drugs these might be, speak with your doctor or pharmacist. This should have been mentioned to you when you started taking one of these medications, but this does not always happen.

3. **IV Lines or Ports**

If you have an IV line or port (this is always the case if you are receiving IV nutrition), then you must be incredibly careful when taking a probiotic and it is often best to avoid them entirely. The risk of getting a blood stream infection from a probiotic when you have an IV line is so high that some probiotic products even carry this warning on their labels. Powders are particularly dangerous, as they will release bacteria into the air, but capsules can also carry residual bacteria on them that may eventually contaminate your line.

We do not have good data right now that would lead us to believe that probiotics will work well for treating the symptoms of digestive disorders or conditions like gastroparesis. There are also some people who would do best to avoid these products completely. However, for the typical, otherwise healthy person, I would not recommend against the use of probiotics as long as you are aware of the possible high cost and the dangers of using a product that is not of high quality.

I cannot stress enough how important it is to be a careful consumer, particularly with probiotics! If you are not able to find one that is third-party certified, call the companies and hold them accountable. If the company is not willing to share information, that is never a good sign. The information that you do receive from them should always indicate that they have checked for contamination from other strains of bacteria before releasing their products to the market. It would be safer and healthier to forego using a probiotic at all than to consider using one that you cannot be certain is not contaminated.

Third-party certified probiotics are not as common as vitamins and minerals, so it may be harder to find a stamp on one of these products.

If you are not able to find one but truly want to use a probiotic, then a call to the company may be appropriate.

Psychiatric Medications

18

In a previous section of this book, we had the opportunity to gain an understanding for the ways that the brain and the GI tract can interact. In fact, we learned that our body actually has two brains, and they communicate in both directions through the brain-gut axis. This provides us with a pathway for exerting some type of control on our symptoms by keeping a handle on our stressors, anxiety, and outlook (see page 74).

This second brain actually provides us with more than just a communication highway from our brains to our guts. In fact, because it is such a dense accumulation of nerves and coordinates its own functions, it has actually been shown to respond to the treatments that we traditionally think of only in relation to use for psychological conditions. Some of the medications that are currently used to treat depression and anxiety have also been shown to have a possibly beneficial impact on the GI symptoms experienced by people with different conditions.

If your doctor suggests one of these treatment options, it does not mean that he thinks your symptoms are all in your head! It actually means that he is attempting to treat your GI condition.

It is important to note that there is a difference between the use of these products for the treatment of a diagnosed psychological condition and for the treatment of GI symptoms. For some people, use of these products will be specifically for clinical depression or anxiety. For others, the use of these products will be specifically for the treatment of GI symptoms. And some people might be killing two birds with one stone – treating both psychological and GI symptoms with only one treatment. We will discuss the implications of each of these situations, including the impact that these medications can have on our guts, brains, and other parts of our bodies.

I mentioned previously that IBS seems to have the closest association between mental state and symptom severity (see page 90). Thus, much of the research on the use of psychological medications in the treatment of symptoms has been conducted in this condition. There is little to no information out there regarding the use of these medications specifically for the treatment of gastroparesis–related symptoms. However, that does not mean that these treatments should not be considered for some people with gastroparesis who have not responded to other medications and lifestyle modification. In fact, many doctors are already exploring these options for that purpose, but it should always be considered a last–line option due to the lack of evidence.

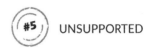

#5 UNSUPPORTED

Use of these medications to treat gastroparesis-related symptoms is not evidence-based at this time. It would be a case of trying to apply information from other conditions in the hope of having a benefit. Thus, these medications are better used for their anxiety and depression treatment properties.

The information that I am going to discuss below will cover the basics of what we know about each of these medications and the effects that they can have throughout the body. When possible, I will point out the medications that have been studied for use in the treatment of GI conditions and for which specific symptoms. Again, using these medications solely to treat gastroparesis–related symptoms is not currently supported by data. However, if you are considering the use of an anti-depressant or antianxiety agent for an existing clinical psychological condition, knowing which options may possibly provide benefit in the GI tract could be helpful. By understanding the pros and cons of each medication, you will be able to have an educated discussion with your physician about whether any of these might be appropriate options for the treatment of your psychological symptoms.

There are a number of different antidepressants on the market. Some of them work in very similar ways, and we will discuss those similar medications as groups, clarifying the differences between the groups instead of each individual drug. An important note that applies to this entire class of medications is that these drugs can take about 6–8 weeks to exert an effect and provide a benefit. During these 6–8 weeks, the side effects from the drug will become apparent. Because of the presence of side effects but the long delay in benefit, some people become discouraged and discontinue use. It is very important to stay the course as long as the side effects are tolerable in order to evaluate whether or not these medications are working for you.

A trial of a new antidepressant must be at least 2-3 months to really see a benefit. This can be a discouraging wait, especially because side effects will appear within this time frame. But if the side effects are tolerable, pushing through the waiting period will allow you the chance of a possible benefit.

There is another consideration that must be made with the use of any antidepressants. The FDA required that all of these products hold a Black Box Warning that states that there is a potentially increased risk for suicidal thoughts and activities when these medications are first started. As the person using these medications, it is very important to be aware of this and the fact that it might happen to you. Although this risk should disappear with continued use, this can be a very dangerous initial side effect.

Finally, antidepressants should never be discontinued abruptly. This can result in withdrawal that can lead to very uncomfortable physical symptoms. Instead, any discontinuation should be discussed with your physician, and a plan to slowly wean you off of the medication should be created.

SELECTIVE SEROTONIN REUPTAKE INHIBITORS (SSRI)
FLUOXETINE (PROZAC), SERTRALINE (ZOLOFT), PAROXETINE (PAXIL), CITALOPRAM (CELEXA), ESCITALOPRAM (LEXAPRO)

This is the most popular class of antidepressants, made famous by the approval of Prozac in 1987.

Since that time, a number of other medications have been developed and approved that fall into this same class, many of which are now quite recognizable due to advertising campaigns.

The SSRIs work by keeping serotonin in the area where it can be used to impact the function of nerve cells. When the drug is not present, serotonin is typically collected back up by a specific cell, and these drugs prevent this from happening. It appears that extended use of SSRIs over time begins to actually change the way that the nerve cells function in relation to serotonin. This change in function also seems to be involved in the antidepressant activity of these medications.

The side effects that occur with these medications are slightly different for each one. In fact, your doctor might suggest a specific option for which the side effects make more sense in your life. The most common GI side effects that are seen with this class are diarrhea, weight loss, and nausea. The other most common side effects are insomnia, drowsiness, headache, night sweats, agitation, and sexual dysfunction. Most psychiatric medications have some type of impact on sleep patterns, either by causing insomnia or by causing drowsiness. An approach that helps to offset this for some people is to take the medication at a different time of day – in the morning if it causes insomnia, at bedtime if it causes drowsiness.

These medications seem to be quite effective for many people in the treatment of clinical depression, anxiety, and other conditions such as obsessive-compulsive disorder (OCD). Benefiting from improvements in these conditions may lead to improvement in GI conditions simply through a more positive psychological state and outlook. When studied specifically for the treatment of GI symptoms, however these drugs have had conflicting results in studies and have not been as promising as other medications. Conflicting results mean that one small study will find a small benefit, but another small study will not. This is

SSRI ANTIDEPRESSANT SNAPSHOT

What does it do?
Makes serotonin more available for use by the nerve cells

How often do I take it?
Once a day (at night if it causes drowsiness; in the morning if it causes insomnia)

How soon will it start to work?
Within 6-8 weeks

What are the most common GI side effects?
Diarrhea, weight loss, nausea

What are the most common non-GI side effects?
Insomnia, drowsiness, headache, night sweats, agitation, sexual dysfunction

Are there drug interactions?
Multiple; consult a pharmacist

How does it come?
Tablet, capsule, liquid

Is it safe in pregnancy?
May be unsafe; consider the benefits before continuing use

Is it safe in breastfeeding?
May be unsafe; consider the benefits before continuing use

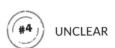 UNCLEAR

why we often need larger groups in order to really understand whether a treatment leads to a certain effect.

This class of medications has been studied during pregnancy and there are some possible concerns to consider if you feel that it is necessary to continue taking an antidepressant in pregnancy. Some studies have shown a possible increased risk for malformations and autism, although the certainty of this association is unclear. Additionally, the use of the medication immediately prior to delivery has resulted in some delivery complications that might be avoided if the medication is discontinued prior to labor under the guidance of a physician. Similarly, there may be risk for side effects such as colic and irritability if these medications are used while breastfeeding. Some of these medications remain in the milk for a shorter time period, so you can speak with your doctor about which options might be best in this situation.

SSRIs are all available as tablets and pills, and many are also available in liquid forms. A few of these medications do have a number of drug interactions, so it important to speak with your pharmacist about anything else that you are taking. If the primary goal of using this medication is to treat GI symptoms, other options should be considered. However, this class of medications has been used successfully for years in the treatment of depression and anxiety, and should be considered if this is your goal with use.

TRICYCLICS
AMITRIPTYLINE (ELAVIL), NORTRIPTYLINE (PAMELOR), IMIPRAMINE (TOFRANIL), DOXEPIN (ZONALON)

These are actually the oldest antidepressants on the market, and they get their name from the structure of the molecules that make up these drugs. These medications seem to have multiple effects on the brain through modulation of both serotonin and norepinephrine, but the exact way that they work is unclear. Tricyclics are not commonly used for the treatment of depression because many of the other medications that we now have available seem to work at least as well and have fewer side effects. The most common GI side effects seen with this group of medications are nausea, significant constipation, and weight gain. Additional side effects include sedation, headache, dry mouth and eyes, and sexual dysfunction. The sedation with these drugs is so significant that most people have to take them at bedtime in order to function during the day. You may remember these medications from our discussion of medications that impact the GI tract – the constipation that is seen here is actually a result of these medications slowing GI motility (see page 60). This is something that should be considered before using in gastroparesis.

When used for purposes other than depression, tricyclics appear to be effective at much lower doses. These lower doses mean that the side effects that come with these drugs are also reduced. One of the most common uses of these medications is in the treatment of nerve pain, a very specific type of pain. They are also growing in popularity for the treatment of GI symptoms seen with both IBS and IBD. Studies have shown that they could be possibly beneficial for reducing loose stools, decreasing the sense of urgency, and also reducing abdominal pain in IBS. Some studies in IBD have also shown that they helped with symptom control. While this is promising, we still need more studies to truly understand when tricyclics can be most beneficial for treating GI symptoms.

Tricyclic use during pregnancy has been shown to cause withdrawal symptoms in newborn babies. Some studies have also indicated the potential for adverse outcomes, such as developmental delays and lung function, but other studies have failed to find this association. Thus, mothers should seriously consider the need to continue this medication during pregnancy against the potential for risks to the baby. Use of these medications in breastfeeding may be relatively safe because only a small amount of the drug transfers into breastmilk. However, this safety has not been fully confirmed, so careful consideration should be made regarding the need for the medication while breastfeeding.

Tricyclics are available in tablets and capsules. Although not many, there are some possible drug interactions with this class, so speak with your pharmacist about your other medications. Dose adjustments are often required to get the treatment right with these drugs. This can take a long time to perfect because each new dose needs to be tested for 6–8 weeks in order to clearly see the benefits and risks before attempting a new dose adjustment or deciding to remain at the current dose.

SEROTONIN-NOREPINEPHRINE REUPTAKE INHIBITORS (SNRI)
DULOXETINE (CYMBALTA), VENLAFAXINE (EFFEXOR), DESVENLAFAXINE (PRISTIQ)

SNRI ANTIDEPRESSANT SNAPSHOT

What does it do?
Makes serotonin and norepinephrine more available for use by the nerve cells

How often do I take it?
Once a day (at night if it causes drowsiness; in the morning if it causes insomnia)

How soon will it start to work?
Within 6-8 weeks

What are the most common GI side effects?
Nausea, constipation, loss of appetite

What are the most common non-GI side effects?
Agitation, dizziness, drowsiness, headache, insomnia, dry mouth

Are there drug interactions?
Multiple; consult a pharmacist

How does it come?
Tablet, capsule

Is it safe in pregnancy?
May be unsafe; consider the benefits before continuing use

Is it safe in breastfeeding?
May be unsafe; consider the benefits before continuing use

Whereas the SSRIs work by keeping serotonin in the area where it can be most utilized for nerve function, the SNRIs work by exhibiting this impact on both serotonin and norepinephrine. This means that their function is closer in nature to the function of the tricyclic family. And, not surprisingly, these medications appear to be beneficial in the treatment of nerve pain, just as is the case with tricyclics.

The most common GI side effects seen with the SNRIs are nausea, constipation, and loss of appetite. Appetite loss could be of concern in someone with gastroparesis, in which it is already difficult to eat consistently and some people have trouble maintaining a healthy interest in food. The other most common side effects for these medications are agitation, dizziness, drowsiness, headache, insomnia, and dry mouth. The occurrence of these side effects is different for each medication in this class, which can help to guide selection of the appropriate drug. For GI indications, a lower dose can be utilized, which may reduce some of the side effects that have been seen with this class of medications.

Although SNRIs are becoming more commonly prescribed for use in GI conditions, very few studies have actually evaluated the use of these medications in IBS. For the studies that are available, a possible improvement was seen in feelings of urgency, as well as abdominal pain. This effect was particularly prominent in people with anxiety. However, the side effects of nausea and reduced appetite were significant concerns for many of these people. More studies are needed before this can be considered a go-to treatment option for GI conditions.

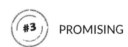 PROMISING

These medications are available as tablets and capsules. There are a small number of drug interactions that can occur, so speak with a pharmacist about anything else that you are taking. The concerns with the use of SNRIs during pregnancy mirror the concerns that are present for SSRIs and tricyclics. The manufacturers of venlafaxine and desvenlafaxine recommend to either discontinue the medication or forego breastfeeding. However, small studies indicate that they may not be as risky as originally thought. Thus, for all of the medications in this class a careful decision should be made considering possible risks to the baby from exposure.

ANTIANXIETY MEDICATIONS

Unlike the medications used to treat depression, the medications used to treat anxiety do not exhibit as many side effects and do not carry an increased risk for suicidal thoughts and actions at the beginning of therapy.

The most famous class of medications that is used to treat anxiety is the benzodiazepines. This class includes very recognizable names, such as Xanax, Valium, and Klonopin. These medications are typically taken when they are needed to control a specific episode of anxiety or to calm frayed nerves. All of the drugs in this class cause impairment of

Benzodiazepines are the classic drugs that people think of for treating anxiety. However, they don't prevent anything - they only work in the moment.

To take control of the brain-gut axis, we must improve mental outlook and reduce stress, so we need to focus on prevention.

mental function and drowsiness, which means that they are not viable options for regular use throughout the day on a consistent basis. Because they do not prevent and control anxiety, I am not going to discuss them in detail here.

Instead we will focus on two specific medications – mirtazapine and buspirone. These two medications are similar to antidepressants in the sense that they are taken every day to help control and prevent the symptoms of anxiety. In fact, some of the antidepressants that we already discussed have been shown to be helpful in the treatment of anxiety as well, and as you will see, the function of these drugs overlap quite a bit.

MIRTAZAPINE (REMERON)

This medication is actually an antidepressant as well as an antianxiety treatment. In fact, it is a great option for people that have both depression and anxiety. It is also used for people who experience sleep disruptions in relation to either of these conditions because it seems to improve sleep patterns. Mirtazapine works in a unique way and does not fall into any other existing antidepressant classes. While it modulates serotonin and norepinephrine activity, it does not work in the same way as SSRIs or SNRIs. It also appears to have at least some activity on other molecules, including histamine and dopamine.

This medication is lacking in many of the side effects that are common amongst the antidepressants that we already discussed. The most common GI side effects with this medication are constipation and increased appetite, which can obviously also lead to weight gain. Surprisingly, mirtazapine actually appears to reduce nausea instead of increase it. Other common side effects include sedation and dry mouth. This sedation lends to a positive impact on sleep when it is taken at bedtime.

Another feature that makes this medication somewhat unusual is that it begins to work more quickly

MIRTAZAPINE SNAPSHOT

What does it do?
Modulates serotonin and norepinephrine activity

How often do I take it?
Once daily at night

How soon will it start to work?
Within 2-3 weeks

What are the most common GI side effects?
Constipation, increased appetite

What are the most common non-GI side effects?
Sedation, dry mouth

Are there drug interactions?
Multiple; consult a pharmacist

How does it come?
Tablet, orally-disintegrating tablet

Is it safe in pregnancy?
May increase risk of miscarriage or early delivery; consider benefits before continuing use

Is it safe in breastfeeding?
Likely safe

than any of the other medications that we have discussed. Its effect can actually be seen as soon as 2 weeks, which means that changes to doses can be made more quickly and you can appreciate the benefits of the medication more rapidly.

There is currently a lack of studies that have really evaluated the use of mirtazapine for the treatment of GI conditions, although it could theoretically be a promising option. There have been a number of case reports indicating improvement in a handful of people, but these should be considered as nothing more than anecdotes until we have more information available to us. Regardless, this may be a great treatment option for people that are experiencing chronic anxiety, or anxiety with depression.

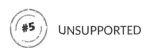 UNSUPPORTED

This medication is available as both a tablet and an orally-disintegrating tablet (how unusual!). There is the potential for a number of interactions with this medication, so speak with a pharmacist about anything else that you are taking. When mirtazapine is used in pregnancy, there is an unclear but possible risk for spontaneous miscarriage and early delivery. Due to this potential, the mother should make a careful decision about the importance of continuing the medication during pregnancy. It appears that only very small amounts of the medication are transferred in breastmilk, so it is likely safe to use while breastfeeding, but this has not been confirmed.

BUSPIRONE (BUSPAR)

Unlike mirtazapine, this medication is only used for the treatment and prevention of chronic anxiety. It works by modulating serotonin at one specific receptor. You might remember that we discussed a group of nausea medications that work on one serotonin receptor – 5HT3 (see page 199). This medication works on another serotonin receptor, specifically 5-HT1A. Serotonin is a surprisingly abundant and multi-talented molecule, with a hand in all kinds of bodily functions! Buspirone is the only antianxiety medication on the market

What does it do?
Modulates serotonin at 5-HT1A

How often do I take it?
Once daily (at night if it causes drowsiness)

How soon will it start to work?
Within 3-6 weeks

What are the most common GI side effects?
Nausea, diarrhea

What are the most common non-GI side effects?
Dizziness, headache, drowsiness

Are there drug interactions?
Multiple; consult a pharmacist

How does it come?
Tablet

Is it safe in pregnancy?
Likely safe

Is it safe in breastfeeding?
Probably safe but there is not enough data to be certain

UNCLEAR (#4)

that does not cause impaired mental function and drowsiness, the biggest issues with the benzodiazepines that were mentioned previously.

When buspirone works in the treatment of anxiety, it works quite well. Unfortunately, there are many people that do not experience a benefit with use. However, this medication generally has very few side effects, making it an appealing option to try even if it does not result in the desired benefit after all. The most common GI side effects seen with buspirone are nausea and diarrhea. Other side effects are dizziness, headaches, and drowsiness. It may take 2 weeks to begin to notice an effect with buspirone, and the drug must be continued for at least 3-6 weeks to notice the full effect. At this time, the dose can be altered if the benefit is inadequate, but the change must be continued for at least 3 weeks to really evaluate it.

A small number of studies have looked at the usefulness of this medication in treating IBS symptoms, but there seems to be some conflicting information. While it looks promising and seems to lead to a benefit for some people, it also appeared to cause more GI side effects in other people, which nullified any benefit that they received. It is clear that more information is needed before buspirone should be used for this reason. However, treating anxiety can be crucial in controlling signals sent down the brain-gut axis, so this medication is a real option for anyone experiencing chronic anxiety.

Buspirone is available as a tablet. There are a number of possible drug interactions with this medication, so speak with a pharmacist about the other drugs that you are taking. With the limited information that is available, buspirone appears to be safe for use during pregnancy. It does not appear that this medication is transferred into breastmilk, but this has not been confirmed. Because it is unclear if it is safe while breastfeeding, a mother should carefully consider the benefit of the medication against possible unknown risks to the baby.

Sleep Disturbances 19

Sleep disturbances are not isolated to those of us with gastroparesis. They are a relatively common occurrence across the general population, and can happen for a number of reasons. For the purposes of this book, we will focus on the two main types of sleep disturbances that fall into the category of insomnia. The first is an inability to fall asleep and the second is an inability to stay asleep, or a tendency to wake up periodically, disrupting the sleep cycle and inhibiting continued rest.

IDENTIFYING THE CAUSE

The most important step in treating insomnia is to identify why it is happening. Sometimes finding the cause can show you a clear solution that can be quickly addressed. For instance, if there is an issue with your surroundings such as noise or light, these can be taken care of through methods like the use of blackout curtains or white noise machines. Similarly, postural discomfort could be managed through the use of a different pillow, mattress, or possibly a mattress topper.

It sounds cliche, but most sleep disturbances can actually be fixed with some minor tweaks to habits and lifestyle, no medication required.

For those with gastroparesis, it may be difficult to fall asleep due to discomfort from GI symptoms. It might be possible to reduce this occurrence by altering your habits. If certain foods consistently cause issues, avoid them at night. If your stomach feels full and painful for a few hours after eating, attempt to eat as far from your intended bedtime as possible. Acid reflux can also be a source of discomfort at bedtime. Propping your head with a stack of pillows can be helpful, as can the use of antacids prior to going to bed.

There are also some general considerations that are commonly associated with insomnia of which every person should be aware. Drinking large amounts of caffeine within 3-4 hours of going to bed can cause issues. Vigorous physical activity or performing tasks that require great mental concentration can also make it difficult to sleep for 1-2 hours after completion. Behavioral conditioning may also be helpful in encouraging our bodies to fall asleep in certain places and at certain times. Keeping a regular schedule is an example of this. Another example would be to not use your bed for anything other than sleeping and restrict your reading and computing activities to a different location entirely.

There are plenty of resources out there that provide guidance for how to manage sleep disturbances without the use of medications. As you can imagine, non-medication interventions are always the best way to address these concerns. Sleep medications are imperfect solutions at best, and many of them have concerning side effects. Lifestyle and behavioral changes should always be made prior to escalating to additional treatments.

IRON DEFICIENCY

We discussed iron previously in our section on nutrient supplementation (see page 145). In that section, we looked at the various ways to correct an iron deficiency, which includes the use of supplements, eating meats, and supplementing iron-rich vegetables with vitamin C. The standard symptom that people associate with iron deficiency is anemia. This anemia leads to a reduction of oxygen transport to our cells, which then results in a general fatigue.

So you may be asking why iron deficiency would be related to sleep disturbances if it is supposed to make us more tired. One of the less commonly recognized complications of iron deficiency is actually restless leg syndrome (RLS). This is a condition in which the legs move and kick involuntarily at night. This involuntary movement can actually be strong enough to wake someone up and disrupt their sleep. This interrupted sleep can then compound on the fatigue felt from the iron deficiency.

Recognizing and treating an iron deficiency is important whenever it is present. However, this is one more way that it can impact a person's daily life. If you are already aware of having an iron deficiency and have been experiencing interrupted sleep, this might help to serve as an explanation. Replenishment of iron is the only way to correct this symptom. For long-term health and wellbeing, iron replenishment is crucial, as is finding a method that will allow you to maintain your iron levels in the future (see page 145).

OTHER MEDICATIONS

There are many medications that carry side effects which can have an impact on our sleep habits. Some medications cause increased wakefulness, while others might cause drowsiness or sedation. When these side effects are present, they should be used to guide when a medication is taken. If it seems to keep you awake, take it in the morning; if it tends to put you to sleep, take it before bed.

If you have recently started a new medication or changed a dose, don't forget that this might be a possible cause of any new sleep disturbances.

In a similar way, other medications can be used as a way to 'treat' sleep disturbances. If a medication that you need already causes drowsiness, this can possibly be used as a sleep inducer. If you know that you will need to start another medication for a certain reason and some of your options can cause drowsiness, perhaps it would be appropriate to select the option that causes drowsiness and take it before bed.

One of the negative cycles that can develop with medications is one in which we start taking more medications to treat the side effects of other medications!

Do your best to steer clear of this by speaking with your doctor about any other treatment options that you could switch to instead of treating the side effect of what you are on.

That being said, there are still going to be medications that will cause side effects for which changing the time that you take it will not eliminate the impact. Some medications simply cause insomnia and taking them in the morning will not change how they make you feel at night. It is important to try to continue these medications for at least a few weeks to see if this effect wears off or can be countered through lifestyle changes. If it cannot, however, then it is important to speak with your doctor about your alternatives.

MEDICATIONS FOR SLEEP

If changes to your lifestyle, medication regimen, and behaviors do not improve your sleep patterns, then medications can be considered as an option. As with any medications, the impact that delayed emptying can have on absorption should be considered. If a medication needs to be taken a certain time period before you go to sleep, then you may need to increase that time frame to accommodate your delayed emptying. This will need to be tailored to your needs with experience and time.

In our section on nausea medications, we discussed the fact that some over-the-counter nausea medications are also used for sleep (such as diphenhydramine) (see page 197). These may be appropriate options for the rare occurrence of insomnia. However, continued use of these products over time leads to the development of tolerance, and the effect eventually wears off. The following medications are better treatment options for cases of chronic insomnia.

MELATONIN

Melatonin is the only option in this list that is available without a prescription, and is actually something that used to be considered an alternative therapy. It now stands as a great example of an alternative therapy that has become an accepted treatment option in medicine because studies have shown that it is safe and effective for the treatment of insomnia. However, it is important to recognize that it is still a dietary supplement. So if you do purchase this product, make sure that you find one that has third-party certification (see page 119).

Melatonin is a substance that occurs naturally in our bodies, so taking it in pill form supplements this molecule that is already present. Unlike the more traditional prescription sleep medications, melatonin does not work by 'knocking you out'. Within the body, melatonin is involved in the regulation of the sleep cycle. In fact, melatonin supplements appear to be most useful in correcting disrupted sleep cycles, such as those caused by changes in work shifts or jet lag.

This product is typically taken 30-60 minutes before bedtime, but keep in mind that this might not be early enough if you have delayed absorption. It is available as a chewable tablet, as well as a liquid, which might be helpful. There appear to be very few side effects with its use, but it can cause abdominal pain and headache. You should be able to tell if it is working for you within a few days of starting. There are no drug interactions with this product. However, it is considered unsafe for use in both pregnancy and breastfeeding.

RAMELTEON (ROZEREM), TASIMELTEON (HETLIOZ)

These are unique medications that fall into a class of their own. This class impacts sleep cycles by targeting specific melatonin receptors in the body. This is very different than the standard sleep medications that work by inducing sedation. They could almost be thought of as a more refined, targeted version of melatonin. And because they are prescription drugs, there are no concerns about the quality of the product.

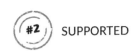 SUPPORTED

MELATONIN SNAPSHOT

What does it do?
Regulates the body's sleep cycle

How often do I take it?
Prior to bedtime

How soon will it start to work?
Within 1 hour

What are the most common side effects?
Abdominal pain, headache

Are there drug interactions?
No

How does it come?
Tablet, chewable, liquid

Is it safe in pregnancy? No

Is it safe in breastfeeding? No

Special Concerns:
This is a dietary supplement, so be sure to find a certified manufacturer

What does it do?
Regulates the body's sleep cycle

How often do I take it?
Prior to bedtime

How soon will it start to work?
Within 1 hour

**What are the most common
side effects?**
Headache, dizziness, nausea

Are there drug interactions?
Multiple; consult a pharmacist

How does it come?
Tablet, capsule

Is it safe in pregnancy? No

Is it safe in breastfeeding?
Possibly safe; breastfeeding
should occur ≥6 hours after dose

Special Concerns:
It may take up to a month to see
the full benefit

Ramelteon and tasimelteon should be taken 30 minutes before bedtime and are only available as tablets or capsules. A high fat meal can make ramelteon less effective, so try to avoid fatty foods within a few hours of taking this medication. There are very few side effects associated with these drugs, but they may cause some dizziness, nausea, and headache. There are a number of possible drug interactions, so make sure to speak with your pharmacist about everything you are taking.

It may take up to a month for these medications to result in their full effect. Both products may be unsafe for use in pregnancy based on birth defects seen when the medications were studied in animals. Safety in breastfeeding is unclear. It is recommended that if a woman chooses to use one of these products while breastfeeding, she allow at least 6 hours to pass after each dose of the medication.

SEDATIVE-HYPNOTICS
ZOLPIDEM (AMBIEN, INTERMEZZO), ZALEPLON (SONATA), ESZOPICLONE (LUNESTA)

These are the most popular sleep treatments and the ones most commonly thought of when sleep medications are discussed. We've all seen the drug ads for these medications and heard some bizarre stories about them on the news. So let's discuss what these drugs actually are and what they can and cannot do.

Each of these medications belong to a class of drugs known as sedative–hypnotics. This means that they induce sleep by binding to certain receptors in the brain called GABA receptors, which helps to cause a sleep state. These medications cause quick sedation and help you to fall asleep very soon after taking them. Their effect is short-lived, however, and will not last throughout the night. This means that if you struggle more with awakening through-out the night than with falling asleep, only a couple of specially formulated options will work for you.

Zolpidem is also available as a controlled-release formulation (Ambien CR), meaning that the drug will be slowly released over time, which allows it to work throughout the night, helping those that often awaken before morning. However, it should be noted that using the controlled-release version of the medication results in a higher chance for sedation and fatigue that can extend into your morning. There is also a special formulation of this drug, branded as Intermezzo, that was specifically designed to be used when people wake up in the middle of the night. It is an orally-disintegrating tablet which can be taken if you awake in the middle of the night and have more than 4 hours left before you plan to get up in the morning.

The most common side effects seen with this group of medications is dizziness and headache. Some people also report memory impairment the next morning and mild hallucinations. These drugs have become quite famous for the news stories on people who have started performing regular activities in their sleep, such as driving, cleaning, cooking, and eating. These side effects are quite unusual, but it would be wise to use these medications initially with someone else in the house to evaluate whether you are susceptible to these risks. While some sleep activities may not be concerning, it is obviously a risk to yourself and others to participate in activities such as sleep driving, and in these cases, the medication should be stopped.

Lunesta and Sonata are available as tablets. The drug that is in Ambien, however, comes in a variety of formulations, including sublingual tablets, orally-disintegrating tablets, and an oral spray. Each of these versions are actually absorbed in the mouth and might be a great alternative for those of you that experience delays in drug absorption from your stomach. A number of drug interactions do exist with these medications, so be sure to speak with your pharmacist about anything else that you are taking.

SEDATIVE-HYPNOTIC SNAPSHOT

What does it do?
Induces a sedated sleep state

How often do I take it?
Prior to bedtime

How soon will it start to work?
Within 1 hour

What are the most common side effects?
Headache, dizziness

Are there drug interactions?
Multiple; consult a pharmacist

How does it come?
Tablet, oral spray, sublingual tablet, orally-disintegrating tablet

Is it safe in pregnancy?
Unclear; only use if truly needed; not safe in days prior to delivery

Is it safe in breastfeeding?
Possibly safe; breastfeeding should not occur overnight

Special Concerns:
These medications have been associated with strange sleep behaviors which should be monitored; they can lead to the development of dependence

It is unclear if these medications are safe for use in pregnancy, as there have been no adequate studies in humans. However, it has been established that newborn babies can experience significant respiratory issues if the medication is taken by the mother in the days prior to delivery. Any use during pregnancy should be carefully considered by the mother, weighing unknown risks to the baby against her need for insomnia treatment. These medications are considered likely safe for breastfeeding as long as feeding or pumping does not occur overnight after the medication is taken.

If a medication may lead to the development of dependence in the person using it, it is considered a controlled substance. The classification system is tiered, so medications with higher risk land in a different class than those with lower risk of dependence.

The drugs in this class do carry a risk for developing dependence on their effect and are considered to be a controlled class of medications. I want to reiterate that these medications are not a cure for insomnia or sleep disturbances and do not resolve the underlying cause for such issues. It is always best to make every effort to identify the reason for any sleep disturbance you are experiencing before using these medications or becoming dependent on their effects.

Female Hormones

20

While it made sense to include this section based solely off of the fact that birth control is the most common medication taken by women, there are actually some distinct ways in which female hormones and gastroparesis interact. Many women with gastroparesis begin to notice an association between their gastroparesis symptoms and their menstrual cycles. Others may begin to notice that their cycles have become more irregular since diagnosis, even while taking birth control. This section will tackle the reasons behind both of these topics and ways to manage these changes.

Sorry, men! Consider yourselves lucky that there is no chapter written specifically for you – one less thing to worry about!

MENSTRUAL CYCLE

In order to have a useful conversation about the impact of female hormones on gastroparesis, we are going to complete a very brief overview of the menstrual cycle and the terms associated with it. The hormones that are responsible for directing this cycle are luteinizing hormone (LH) and follicle-stimulating hormone (FSH). These hormones stimulate the body to produce estrogen and progesterone. There are three phases to this cycle:

1. **Follicular phase**

   This stage starts with menstruation and ends with the release of the egg. It typically lasts about 11–14 days, but will vary for each woman.

2. **Ovulatory phase**

   This is the stage in which the egg is released, and only lasts for about 16–32 hours.

3. **Luteal phase**

   This stage occurs after ovulation and involves preparation for a fertilized egg to implant on the wall of the uterus.

Menstrual Cycle Phases and Hormones

Follicular Phase: Follicle-stimulating hormone and estrogen

Ovulatory Phase: Luteinizing hormone

Luteal Phase: Progesterone

In the luteal phase, a high level of progesterone is produced to thicken the uterine wall and allow for a fertilized egg to implant. If an egg does not implant, then the endometrial tissue begins to shed, resulting in what we know as menstruation. In the resulting follicular phase, the body begins to produce FSH and estrogen to prepare an egg for ovulation. During ovulation, the level of LH becomes very high.

Stated very simply, birth control impacts this cycle by regulating the amount of estrogen and progesterone that are present at any given time. This prevents an egg from being released during ovulation, and it also makes the mucus in the cervix stickier, which limits the amount of sperm that can get through.

While that was indeed a brief overview, that is all we need in order to talk about the ways that female hormones and gastroparesis can overlap. We will use the terms for the hormones and phases that are involved in the cycle during this section.

GASTROPARESIS AND THE MENSTRUAL CYCLE

Believe it or not, there have been studies conducted to look specifically at gastric emptying during the menstrual cycle, as well as whether or not women experience worsened symptoms from gastroparesis at different points in their cycles. We will take a look at both of these concepts.

First, a study was conducted that compared the gastric emptying times for healthy women to that of healthy men. While they found that women had slightly delayed emptying in comparison to men, this finding is already generally understood in the medical community. They also looked for a difference in the gastric emptying times for women in the luteal phase and in the follicular phase.

Women have slightly slower gastric emptying than men on a normal day.

They did not find a difference in emptying times at different phases of the menstrual cycle. This study was not conducted in people that already had gastroparesis, so we cannot be certain if hormonal changes may have a different impact in someone who already has delayed emptying. However, this study seems to indicate that our emptying times do not appear to actually change during various stages of the menstrual cycle.

A different study was conducted to evaluate symptoms for women with gastroparesis at different points in their menstrual cycles and compare symptoms for those that were or were not taking birth control. This study surveyed 20 women that were not taking birth control (half with gastroparesis, half without) and 20 women that were taking birth control (half with gastroparesis, half without). They asked each woman extensive questions throughout her entire menstrual cycle and compared the reported symptoms.

The evaluation found that women not taking birth control had worsened symptoms during the luteal phase than during the follicular phase in comparison to those taking birth control. These worsened symptoms included nausea and feelings of fullness. In general, women with gastroparesis that were not taking birth control had noticeable fluctuations in the experience of symptoms. The women with gastroparesis that were taking birth control did not experience increased symptoms during the luteal phase, and also appeared to have more stable day-to-day symptoms throughout the duration of a menstrual cycle.

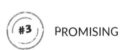

#3 PROMISING

RESULTS

Not on birth control:

More symptom fluctuation
More nausea and fullness
  during the luteal phase

On birth control:

More stable symptoms
No changes within cycle

This study indicates that younger women with gastroparesis should consider the use of birth control for the purposes of regulating symptom fluctuations and reducing the increase in certain symptoms that may occur for some people. Whenever possible, the birth control that is selected should be a low-dose option. This is due to the fact that estrogen and progesterone are known to cause stomach discomfort. In addition, other studies have indicated that these hormones may have some type of impact on stomach emptying, although the significance is unclear.

While many women can safely use birth control, there are some for which this is not a good idea. For example, many birth control products have the potential to increase a woman's risk of developing a blood clot. This risk is higher in women that have a history of a blood clot, are very overweight, or that smoke cigarettes, so these women should only use certain forms of birth control. Please discuss your full medical history with your doctor prior to initiating birth control to make sure that it is the right choice for you.

BIRTH CONTROL

We have already discussed the ways that gastroparesis can impact the passage and absorption of medications within the GI tract (see page 58). Hormone products are no different. Their absorption can be both delayed and reduced, depending on the situation and the severity of each person's condition.

Many of you are probably aware that your birth control products must be taken at the same time every day. In fact, a lot of women even set an alarm to remind them to take it daily, on schedule. So what happens when you take it on time, but then it sits in your stomach for hours on end or moves very slowly through your intestine? Or what if you vomit it back up because it causes additional nausea? You could cross your fingers and hope that it experiences the same delay every day, which means that it is being absorbed around the same time every day. But we all know how variable our symptoms can be depending on what we have eaten, what else we might be sick with, and also whether we are experiencing a flare.

No matter what you are taking birth control for, whether it be to regulate an irregular cycle and/or your gastroparesis symptoms, to reduce debilitating cramps and bleeding, or to prevent pregnancy, you do not want to risk inappropriate absorption of this medication. Experiencing more cycles, or more painful cycles, only stands to exacerbate your gastroparesis and lower your quality of life as we just discussed. Accidentally becoming pregnant is an entirely different, and very large, concern.

Fortunately for us, there are actually a growing number of alternative forms of birth control being developed. This means that you don't necessarily have to take a pill. In fact, there are shots, patches, vaginal rings, and most recently, an implant. All of these are in addition to the long–term contraceptive option, the intrauterine device (IUD). We'll briefly discuss each of these options and their different pros and cons here. Each one represents an alternative that would allow you to avoid the uncertain effect of an oral medication and also the possible stomach upset that it can cause.

INJECTION
(DEPO-PROVERA, MEDROXYPROGESTERONE)

The birth control injection has actually been an option for a few decades, so most of you are already probably familiar with the concept. It is an injection that is placed into the arm muscle once every 3 months. The reason that it can be done so infrequently is that the injection itself is formulated in a way that causes the drug to slowly release from the muscle and into the body over that 3–month time frame.

One of the things about this injection that concerns some women is the fact that it prevents consistent periods. Additionally, it is known to cause

BIRTH CONTROL INJECTION SNAPSHOT

How often do I take it?
Once every 3 months

How soon will it start to work?
Immediately

What are the most common side effects?
Spotting, loss of regular periods

Are there major side effects?
There is a possibility for loss of bone density with extended use

What benefits are there?
Protection against endometrial cancer; helpful in endometriosis

Is it safe in pregnancy? No

Is it safe in breastfeeding? Yes

spotting and bleeding, which means that not only will you not have a regular period, you will bleed at unexpected times. This tends to level out after the first few months of use, but it is a deterrent for some women. Another concern that used to exist with this product was additional weight gain, but further research has clarified that the weight gain with this injection is no different than for women taking the pill.

A unique trait of this injection is that it contains only progesterone, whereas the large majority of birth control options contain estrogen as well. This is a great option for women that cannot utilize estrogen for any reason. It also lends to an apparent protective effect against endometrial cancer and may be beneficial for women with endometriosis. There is a concern that it can cause bones to become more frail with use over a long period of time, but no studies have confirmed how significant this is, and it also appears to be reversible when the medication is stopped. This is of greatest concern for younger women who have not yet reached peak bone mass.

The injection offers a real alternative to the pill and may be particularly advantageous for a certain group of women. However, there are many other options out there that are typically preferred over the injection.

PATCH
(ORTHO EVRA, XULANE)

The birth control patch has been around for quite some time. It was very exciting when it was first released, and many women were looking forward to the option to ditch a daily pill and start applying a patch. The patch is applied for 3 weeks and then removed for 1 week.

Although it might seem counterintuitive, women actually experience a number of the side effects that are seen with the pill, including nausea and breast tenderness and swelling. The patch has also been

BIRTH CONTROL PATCH SNAPSHOT

How often do I take it?
Apply once a month

How soon will it start to work?
Immediately

What are the most common side effects?
Nausea, breast tenderness and swelling

Are there major side effects?
This carries the highest risk of blood clotting

What benefits are there?
Standard for birth control

Is it safe in pregnancy? No

Is it safe in breastfeeding?
Not recommended for 21 days after delivery; there are small risks to the baby so consider the need for use while breastfeeding

shown to cause skin irritation in a small number of the women that use it. Every birth control that contains estrogen has the potential to increase a woman's risk of developing a blood clot. However, the patch actually appears to carry an even higher risk for clot than other available forms of birth control.

While the patch may be an appropriate choice for some women, there are possibly better options that can be considered in order to avoid the increased nausea and risk of blood clots.

RING
(NUVARING)

The vaginal ring is a very unique form of birth control that is inserted into the vagina once a month and then removed after 3 weeks. This ring releases hormones slowly during that entire time frame. However, it does not appear to have the increased risk for blood clots that is seen with the patch. Instead, it seems to have the same risk as the pill.

The ring has been compared directly to the use of the patch and has shown a significant reduction in nausea, as well as breast swelling and pain. It also led to a reduction in the heaviness of bleeding and the duration of bleeding in comparison to the patch and the pill. The only side effect that was actually seen to be higher with the use of the ring was an increase in vaginal discharge. While the ring cannot be felt while it is placed in the vagina, it can sometimes push itself back out, which is a strange sensation and somewhat of a nuisance. It may also be felt by a partner during intercourse, but this is typically not a deterrent for women that use it.

In fact, in studies that compared the ring to any other birth control options, the ring was consistently the preferred option and was more likely to be recommended to friends. The largest potential downside to the ring in comparison to other options is its price. Through the Affordable Care

BIRTH CONTROL RING SNAPSHOT

How often do I take it?
Insert once a month

How soon will it start to work?
Immediately

What are the most common side effects?
Increased vaginal discharge

Are there major side effects?
No

What benefits are there?
Reduction in bleeding heaviness and duration

Is it safe in pregnancy? No

Is it safe in breastfeeding?
Not recommended for 21 days after delivery; there are small risks to the baby so consider the need for use while breastfeeding

Act, all insurance plans are required to cover birth control at no charge, which effectively renders this concern irrelevant. A small number of religious healthcare plans, however, are exempted from this requirement. If you are on a plan that does not cover birth control due to religious reasons, speak with your doctor about obtaining a special authorization. Because of your gastroparesis, you are able to claim a legitimate medical need for using birth control that is not related to the prevention of pregnancy.

IMPLANT
(IMPLANON, NEXPLANON)

BIRTH CONTROL IMPLANT SNAPSHOT

How often do I take it?
Placed once every 3 years

How soon will it start to work?
Immediately

What are the most common side effects?
Spotting, loss of regular periods

Are there major side effects?
No

What benefits are there?
Protection against endometrial cancer; helpful in endometriosis

Is it safe in pregnancy? No

Is it safe in breastfeeding? Yes

The birth control implant has actually been available in the United States since 2006 but is still not commonly heard about or talked about. It is basically a tiny stick that is placed under the skin and remains there for up to 3 years. It slowly releases hormones from that location over time.

This is a great option for basically any woman that is a candidate for birth control. Much like the injection, this is also a product that contains only progesterone. This means that it does not carry an increased risk for blood clots. It also means that it might yield some protective benefits against endometrial cancer and also appears to be a good option for women with pain associated with endometriosis. Unlike the injection, there does not appear to be an increased risk for reduction in bone density with the implant.

The most common side effect noted by women with the use of this implant was irregular bleeding, much like what is seen with the injection. However, the injection causes a woman's period to stop, whereas the implant does not. It appears that the irregular bleeding slowly reduces after a few months of having the implant and may become more manageable at that time.

It is worth nothing that removal of the implant, while typically a non-issue, can cause soreness, pain, and scarring for some women depending on how deeply it was placed under the skin. Speak with your doctor regarding their level of experience with the product and what you should expect.

INTRAUTERINE DEVICES - IUDS
(PARAGARD, MIRENA)

IUDs have somewhat of a tarnished history in the United States due to what was originally a poor understanding for appropriate use and appropriate implantation. However, the past 20-30 years have seen great success with these products and provided us quite a bit of information that is reassuring regarding their safety and efficacy.

IUDs, as the term would indicate, are actually small devices that are implanted into the uterus for extended periods of time. There are two types of IUDs currently available. The version that most people think of when they hear the term IUD is the copper product, which can be implanted for up to 10 years. The newer IUD actually contains levonorgestrel, a form of progesterone, and it can be implanted for up to 5 years.

Most women are good candidates for the use of an IUD if they want a very long-term solution to birth control and do not intend to have children in the next 5-10 years. Some of the original concerns with IUDs centered around possible infection risk or damage that could result in infertility. Now that we have many years of data available, it appears that there is no risk of infertility and the only risk for infection is a small risk that occurs immediately after implantation of the device. IUDs can also be great options for women that cannot take estrogen or are at an increased risk for blood clotting.

The copper and levonorgestrel devices have opposite effects on the menstrual cycle. The copper IUD may lead to heavier and longer periods, particularly in the first few months after placement. Women will continue to have a period on a monthly basis when they are using this product. The levonorgestrel

---

COPPER IUD SNAPSHOT

How often do I take it?
Placed once every 10 years

How soon will it start to work?
Immediately

What are the most common side effects?
Heavier, longer periods

Are there major side effects?
No

What benefits are there?
Non-hormonal, but this means that it will not lead to regulation of symptoms or cycle

Is it safe in pregnancy? No

Is it safe in breastfeeding? Yes

LEVONORGESTREL IUD SNAPSHOT

How often do I take it?
Placed once every 5 years

How soon will it start to work?
Immediately

What are the most common side effects?
Spotting, loss of regular periods

Are there major side effects?
No

What benefits are there?
Protection against endometrial cancer; helpful in endometriosis

Is it safe in pregnancy? No

Is it safe in breastfeeding? Yes

IUD, on the other hand, causes many of the effects that are seen with the birth control injection, as they are both progesterone-only products. It may lead to a discontinuation of periods for up to 20% of women that use it and may also increase the occurrence of random spotting and bleeding. For women that are currently experiencing heavy or painful periods, this device appears to have a positive impact on both the heaviness and pain involved in menstruation, and it may provide protection against endometrial cancer.

I think it is very important to point out that the benefit of regulating symptoms with gastroparesis may not be present with the use of the copper IUD. This device actually works by interfering with the ability of the sperm to fertilize the egg. It does not regulate hormones or exert any such effect on the menstrual cycle. The levonorgestrel product, however, does provide hormonal regulation, which may lead to some of the desired improvement in GI symptoms from cycle regulation.

CHOOSING THE RIGHT OPTION

There are clearly a wide variety of options out there. Simply by hearing about the different forms, you may have a personal preference as far as comfort and usability. When you read further about additional advantages (ie. for women with endometriosis), one option may become even more appealing. And finally, there may be specific side effects that are particularly troublesome for you. By simply learning about the functionality, pros, and cons of each product, you will probably find yourself favoring one or two of the available options.

Have a discussion with your doctor that includes your full medical history and your future plans. Let your doctor know what your preference is and why. Then you can have an educated and helpful discussion that will narrow down what your best non-oral birth control option might be. If you are transitioning from the pill or actually starting birth control for the first time in hopes that it will help to better regulate your symptoms, make sure that you monitor your symptoms and pay attention for side effects. It can take a few months for some initial side effects with birth control to settle out, at which point you should be able to tell if you are feeling better or worse. If you are feeling worse at that point in time, it might be appropriate to talk to your doctor about switching to a different form.

HORMONE REPLACEMENT THERAPY (HRT)

For women that are entering into menopause, birth control is no longer a concern. Instead, the focus shifts to considerations for replacing the hormones in the body to offset the symptoms that come with menopause.

There are currently no published studies available regarding the topic of HRT and gastroparesis. But it is not a stretch to imagine that if the hormonal shifts in the menstrual cycle can lead to symptomatic changes in gastroparesis, it is possible that the hormonal shifts in menopause can have the same result. During perimenopause, a woman's hormone levels change significantly and fluctuate much more than they do in the postmenopausal stage. After menopause, hormone levels will remain relatively stable, but they will be permanently altered from what was experienced prior to menopause, which may have the potential to result in an overall shift in gastroparesis symptoms.

Menopause:
The ceasing of menstruation

Perimenopause:
The period of life shortly before menopause occurs

You are likely aware of the Women's Health Initiative studies that led to a national scare regarding hormone replacement therapy. People suddenly became very concerned that the extended use of hormone replacement could increase the risk of various issues, from heart disease to breast cancer. Since that time, however, we have gained a better understanding for what does and does not lead to these safety concerns and how to use hormone replacement appropriately.

HRT is recommended by most doctors for many women with perimenopause. Hormone use at this stage can help to reduce a lot of the symptoms that come with this life change, including mood swings, hot flashes, and severe anxiety. However, certain forms of replacement after perimenopause may become more dangerous the longer that they are continued. If you are considering replacement therapy, have a thorough conversation with your doctor about the risks and benefits and how they relate to you specifically. OB GYNs are very knowledgeable on this topic and I would recommend seeing one so that you can have your risks and benefits clearly laid out and explained. Make sure that you let your doctor know that you are concerned about fluctuations in hormones with your gastroparesis.

Since hormone replacement is not used to regulate your menstrual cycle as with birth control, it is not necessary to take these medications at exactly the same time every day. Thus, it is not crucial to consider non-oral options for these medications. These hormones can cause stomach upset, however, so feel free to ask your doctor if one of the patches that are currently available for hormone replacement might be an appropriate option for you.

IN VITRO FERTILIZATION (IVF)

In vitro fertilization:
A complex set of procedures used to treat fertility or genetic problems and assist in conceiving a child

I am including this segment only because I have received so many questions regarding this topic. Unfortunately, no studies have been conducted specifically evaluating in vitro fertilization in gastroparesis. Any guidance that I can provide would be limited to the understanding that IVF requires the use of large doses of hormones, something that could possibly result in gastroparesis symptom fluctuation and flares. If you enter into the IVF process, you should be prepared for this possibility.

I do want to speak a word of caution regarding pregnancy in gastroparesis. Some women do quite well with pregnancy and others do not. Some women find that they feel better during pregnancy but become much sicker afterwards. Each person's experience could be quite different, and you should be aware of the possible outcomes in advance. I am not saying that women with gastroparesis should never become pregnant. In fact, I have specifically included pregnancy and breastfeeding information for all of the medications in this book because pregnancy with gastroparesis is so common.

It is also quite important to be sure that you are at a place in your journey in which it is appropriate to consider pregnancy. Make sure that you are able to consistently maintain your nutritional status and avoid nutrient deficiencies. This will be harder to do during pregnancy, and deficiencies could cause developmental issues for your baby. Having a solid symptom management plan in place will also be crucial to help you handle any ups and downs that you experience with this change in life. Whatever you do, speak openly with your doctor about your plans and that you want to be made aware of any specific concerns that might exist.

Diabetes and Gastroparesis

21

The occurrence of gastroparesis as a result of diabetes is the most common known cause of gastroparesis. Because diabetes requires the close monitoring of blood sugar, there are unique concerns related to diabetic gastroparesis. We will briefly cover some of these concerns and the general approaches to addressing them. It is very important for anyone with both of these conditions to identify a strong medical team. This team must be able to understand your situation and aid in finding creative and simplified ways to manage blood sugar control in the context of gastroparesis.

DIABETES WITH GASTROPARESIS

The development of gastroparesis as a result of diabetes usually occurs only after diabetes has been present for quite some time. In fact, it is often seen in people with Type I diabetes, the form of diabetes that often occurs in childhood and is related to a loss of the cells that create insulin. The development of gastroparesis is a sign that the diabetes may not be well-controlled. There is a possibility that diabetes which remains poorly controlled can lead to a worsening of symptoms and a further delay in emptying times, but this is controversial and has not been proven.

It is also possible for people that already have gastroparesis to develop diabetes at a later point in life. In this case it would be Type II diabetes. This is the form of diabetes that people are often more familiar with, as it is the most common one and occurs as age and weight increase. In fact, the development of this form of diabetes is typically due to the body no longer being able to keep up with its insulin needs, which can be related to both poor diet and increased weight.

Finally, while not actually a form of diabetes, many people with gastroparesis do end up experiencing disturbances in sugar balance. Sometimes large amounts of sugar can be digested at once, or a person could also go for long periods of time without digesting any sugar at all. Either of these occurrences can lead to large hikes or drops in blood sugar levels, and this can cause a variety of symptoms, including shaking, dizziness, sweating, fainting, and more.

Three considerations of blood sugar and gastroparesis:

- Gastroparesis caused by diabetes
- Diabetes that develops in those with gastroparesis
- Sugar absorption fluctuations in those with gastroparesis but no diabetes

Regardless of the situation that you find yourself in, control of blood sugar is incredibly important to long-term health. The complications of poor blood sugar control can be very serious, both for those with diabetes and for those that experience sugar absorption fluctuations.

DIABETES MANAGEMENT WITH GASTROPARESIS

It is a logical conclusion that delays in stomach emptying can make management of blood sugar levels much more difficult, which in turn makes the management of diabetes much more difficult. It is not a bad idea to consider seeing an endocrinologist that specializes in diabetes management. This type of specialty physician is more likely to have creative solutions and ideas, as well as a better understanding for the challenges you are facing, than your general physician.

The delays in stomach emptying that come with gastroparesis will often require a change to a person's current insulin regimen. This change might be related to when you take your insulin. For instance, many people with diabetes take their insulin immediately prior to eating a meal. However, with delayed emptying, it might make more sense to change this practice and take your insulin after you have eaten.

Tighter control of blood sugar can also be obtained through more frequent blood glucose checks after you have eaten. This would allow you to administer insulin more frequently as you see that you need it. However, there are obviously a number of disadvantages to having to do this, including the discomfort and inconvenience of multiple finger sticks and insulin injections. Although it will not be an appropriate option for everyone, many people who are struggling with their management and the increased monitoring that is required may want to speak with their doctors about the use of an insulin pump. This can aid in simplifying and streamlining your blood sugar control under the guidance of an experienced physician.

Carbohydrates are some of the most easily tolerated foods for those with gastroparesis, but they can cause sugar control to become more difficult for those with diabetes.

Speak with a dietician about the benefits of eating whole grains and other forms of carbohydrates along with options such as the insulin pump.

Another change that may be helpful in addition to increased blood glucose checks and insulin administrations is to change the frequency of your meals. Smaller meals spaced out throughout the day may be helpful in regulating the amount of sugar that enters your body over time and eliminate some of the larger delays that can be seen in digestion and emptying. The advice of an experienced diabetes dietician should be sought out regarding this topic. The same dietician may also be able to help in the difficult task of identifying foods that are tolerable with gastroparesis which are not a cause for concern with diabetes.

OTHER INTERVENTIONS

There are a number of medications on the market that are prescribed for the purpose of lowering blood sugar levels in people with diabetes. These may be helpful for some people that struggle with control in relation to their gastroparesis. I will not cover those medications in detail here, but it is important to note that some of the medications on the market for diabetes actually work by slowing down stomach motility. For those without gastroparesis, this reduces appetite and slows the body's absorption of sugars. However, for those with gastroparesis, this can significantly worsen symptoms and make management of your diabetes even more difficult.

The GLP-1 analogues work intentionally to slow stomach emptying, and there are a number of options currently on the market. These include exenatide (Byetta, Burdeon), albiglutide (Tanzeum), dulaglutide (Trulicity), liraglutide (Victoza, Saxenda), and lixisenatide (Adlyxin). Some of these GLP-1 analogues are now also available in combination products with insulin, including Xultophy and LixiLan. A second medication class, the amylin analogues, also intentionally slows stomach emptying, but there is currently only one medication approved in this class - pramlintide (Symlin).

It is important to ensure that you are not currently taking an amylin or GLP-1 analog medication and that your physician does not prescribe one of these products as a way to control your blood sugars. Many other diabetes medications are available that do not cause this increased delay in emptying.

Anyone with gastroparesis that is having a particularly difficult time controlling their diabetes and also consuming adequate calories may benefit from the use of feeding tubes (see page 155). Utilizing these tubes and controlled feeding schedules can help to regulate the digestion and absorption of sugars. While this is never an ideal option and should be considered as more of a last resort, the use of a post-pyloric tube may allow for someone to standardize their insulin administration and requirements, which can help to reduce both stress and sugar imbalances.

General Lifestyle Considerations

22

The second part of this book has been relatively intense with discussions about treatments and medications. Now that we have finished those sections, it's time to lighten up! I wanted to cover some of the general concepts that many of us with gastroparesis have found helpful in making both the condition and the lifestyle changes around it more manageable.

I can't say enough times how important it is to be open to new ideas, mixing things up, and giving yourself a break!

From a worldly point of view, there is no mistake so great as that of being always right.

SAMUEL BUTLER

You will notice that a common theme with all of these general concepts is moderation and practicality. Very few people will be successful in an approach that requires you to do something all of the time, or in an approach that is overly strict and devoid of enjoyable activities and indulgences. We're all human – we need to have fun, break the rules, and enjoy ourselves every once in a while! And in the same way, we need to be allowed to have bad days and setbacks. These will only help us to appreciate the good times even more.

EXERCISE

Find some type of physical activity that works for you. There are endless studies out there that show the extensive mental and physical benefits that can be had from physical activity. Some people will find that going outdoors for this activity is also refreshing. The only rules for your physical activity are that you have to enjoy it and your stomach must be able to tolerate it!

I've spoken about my rediscovered love for walking and hiking. Others with gastroparesis fall in love with biking, because it is low impact and easy on the stomach. Yet others would rather find themselves in a gym, where stationary bikes or elliptical machines can be used for low impact activity. If you're having a really great day, maybe you can try something adventurous, like Zumba or swimming. A physical trainer may be helpful in finding you an activity that you enjoy and tolerate, and they may also be able to provide you very useful guidance on keeping your different muscle groups toned.

There are many claims out there regarding the amount of activity that should be completed every week and whether it should be strenuous or low-level. But the reality is that these recommendations fall all over the place, and for many of us with gastroparesis, getting any activity at all is an improvement. So how about this? Find what works best for you and do it as often as you can. It should be a rewarding cycle of increased activity and improved physical and mental health.

If you find yourself collapsing under the expectations for exercise and instead getting none at all, just throw them out and get yourself moving in some way.

If you find something that you enjoy, you'll find yourself seeking it out as much as possible. And that's a positive cycle that will yield more exercise than most people ever get!

DIET

I really hate the term "diet" because I feel like it implies a temporary change in food intake. But in reality, it refers to everything that we consume. And what we choose to consume can have a pretty big impact on our mental and physical health. When we think of our diet in terms of gastroparesis, we should be thinking of it as a long-term modification to our lifestyle that will make us feel better.

There are obviously a number of nutrition guidelines out there that should be followed as much as possible, but I will defer to a dietician for guidance on those details. You will find that it is easier to follow many of the expectations of these guidelines if you keep a reasonable and metered approach. For instance, if a guideline says to target X grams of fat, just try to get close to that, or average out to that every week.

Make changes in moderation and rely on trial and error. Know that in order to find the foods that you most enjoy and also tolerate, you will have to push through trying some foods that don't make you feel very well at all. Pick a day that makes sense for you to try something new, where you can curl up with a book or in front of the TV and hide away in case it doesn't go well. In the same way, don't restrict yourself to boring and bland foods. You'll find that your mental health goes quickly downhill when your diet is restricted and unenjoyable. If you know that you love a certain food but don't tolerate it well, sneaking a bite or two here and there might actually make you happy and not have a huge impact on your symptoms.

Rethink the reasons that you feel stuck doing certain things. Are the reasons legitimate or applicable to you now? Or can you write some of your own rules?

If you find that you're constantly struggling to comply with social standards or expectations even though your gastroparesis is pushing back, reconsider if you need to be doing that. Breakfast has long been considered a mainstay in our culture. However, recent studies have shown that it does not appear to offer the health benefits that we always thought it did. So if you've been pushing yourself to eat a full breakfast because you "should" but it isn't being tolerated well, maybe you should reconsider. Or if you are trying to eat meals when everyone else does but are experiencing a lot of discomfort and symptoms, maybe you should mix in small meals throughout the day, and take home a bunch of leftovers when you are out with others.

DISTRACTORS

I am going to use this term to broadly include any activities, events, or practices that might act as a distraction from your symptoms. Focusing on how you feel and all of your symptoms will only lead to a magnification of those things. Even when you are not feeling up to doing much, forcing yourself to do something other than think about how you feel is almost always guaranteed to actually make you feel better. There is only one rule to apply – the distractor can't involve food.

Find activities that you really enjoy. I'm a book worm, and when I get into a really good book, the world around me falls away, including what might have been some pretty bad symptoms that day. Other people have this experience with TV shows and movies. Some people will experience this by having conversational social interactions or playing with their kids.

Identify social events that don't involve food, such as concerts, book clubs, sewing groups, etc. You can even consider social events that may have food present but don't require you to consume any in order to fit in, such as sporting events. If you have a hobby that you really enjoyed prior to developing gastroparesis, see if it still makes sense for you now or if there are ways to change it so that it can. Many of us accidentally abandon things that we used to enjoy because we became so caught up in our new condition and symptoms and put aside the things that we love.

Distractors go hand in hand with keeping yourself busy. While it may seem daunting to go to school or work when you are feeling sick, you might find that it is exactly what you need. When our brains are forced to focus on something else, our symptoms suddenly seem less overwhelming. In fact, it is easy to fall into a vicious cycle of working less, feeling worse, and then working even less. If you are in a situation that allows it, challenge yourself to do more and see how you feel. If your work situation won't accommodate that, consider volunteering. Getting yourself moving and distracted would only be augmented by the mental impact that can be obtained from making a difference for others!

Usually the biggest hurdle is convincing yourself to start doing something when you're not feeling well, even if it is just something small like reading or getting up and moving.

But if you can make that first step, you will rarely regret what happens next.

EXPLAINING OR NOT EXPLAINING

Many of us with gastroparesis struggle to decide who we should tell about our conditions and what we should tell them. Having an "invisible" condition cuts both ways. We can skate along without telling anyone unless we absolutely must because there is no obvious sign. However, we are also expected to behave normally and conduct ourselves the way that everyone else would. This may be fine in most situations but becomes more difficult with closer friends, family members, and coworkers.

It is very important to have a small group of people who understand what you are dealing with and that support your needs. Keeping this small group close to you is incredibly valuable to mental health. Beyond that, it is up to each person if they would like to spread the word further, and how much detail they want to provide. I know that I personally don't tell anyone that is not close to me. If a situation arises in which I have to explain something that happened, I try to keep the description brief. I am not personally a fan of being treated differently or being peppered with questions like 'Hey, can you eat this? What about this? Does this bother you?' very often.

Others would never succeed with my approach and even feel a type of acceptance and release in sharing their experiences. Each person is different. You will find what works best for you. I can say from my own experience that if you think you should say something, you probably should. I have kept my mouth shut in many situations and ended up making it more and more awkward as time went on and I tried to find that right moment again.

COMFORT FOODS

Dieticians may snub these but everyone has them. These are the foods that you know will go down easily and make you feel 'better' when you're just not doing well. They act as our go-to's when we are having a flare, or even when we are just experiencing a lot of stress at work or at home.

Sometimes it is wise to turn to comfort foods. If life seems to be throwing you obstacles in every direction, it is probably not the right time to be testing your boundaries and trying new foods. In the same way, it is probably not the right time to be eating foods that may cause you issues. Comfort foods can help to reduce the concerns that you have to deal with in relation to your gastroparesis so that you can focus on everything else that is demanding your attention.

However, it is important not to get yourself into a rut with your food options. If you are turning to your comfort foods, make sure you monitor how much and for how long. Perhaps your stressors and obstacles will die down and you will naturally incorporate more foods back into your daily diet. But if not, you need to have some mechanism in place to break you out of the cycle and make sure you are consuming a varied and healthy diet again.

It may be helpful to develop a way to track ruts in your diet and lifestyle so that you can see when you've fallen into one and pull yourself back out.

COMFORT CLOTHES

At first glance, it might sound like I'm going to talk about the virtues of sweatpants and oversized T-shirts. But, alas, that is not the point in this section. In fact, I want to talk about the clothes that can allow us to feel wholly a part of society and also very comfortable. I am sure many of you have experienced the discomfort of feeling bloated or overweight and wondering if other people can see it because the outfit that you are wearing is a little bit tight. Or maybe you have felt bloated and uncomfortable and your clothes have pushed and prodded in ways that make you feel even worse.

As someone who holds a professional job, I need to dress up for work most of the days that I go in (although sometimes I get to wear scrubs, and I will never complain about that!). In addition, I am not a big fan of wearing sweat pants or pajamas outside of the house. This has forced me to get creative. I want to look good and I also want to feel good. When I'm not worried about my clothes pressuring my stomach or whether anyone can tell how bad I feel, I happen to actually feel better.

I have found that elastic waistband slacks work miracles in making me feel better and hiding any bloating that is occurring (from what I have seen, New York & Co has the largest variety of options). I have also begun to wear more dresses and skirts because they do not apply the same pressure as pants. The maternity section has become a regular stop for me, where I will do a quick once-over to see if there are any nice options that do not actually look like maternity clothes. Every person should try to find a way to make themselves feel good about the way that they look – it really does help to reduce stress and improve outlook.

DRINKS

I have mentioned a few times in this book that I do better with carbonated liquids than still liquids. Others may find that they do better with hot or cold. And yet others might do best with liquids that are in their foods, even in the form of soups. Some people tolerate blended or pureed foods very well whereas others do not. Each person is different and each person will have to find their 'sweet spot' when it comes to consuming food and drink.

One topic that comes up a lot with gastroparesis is whether or not it is OK to drink alcohol. I'll start with my personal experience. I didn't touch the stuff until 2 years after I had my neurostimulator placed. I didn't have any interest in tasting it, re-tasting it, dealing with how it made me feel, or anything else. In addition, alcohol has been shown to slow down stomach emptying in healthy people. All of that being said, I now happily sip on a beer or two (there's that carbonation again!) every few days. I don't find that my stomach empties at a noticeably slower rate. And what I do notice is that a small amount of alcohol every few days keeps me in a more positive place mentally.

Some interesting research in recent years has shown that people who consume 1-2 alcoholic beverages every couple of days may actually live longer than people that drink no alcohol at all. This is possibly related to the stress and anxiety reduction that small amounts of alcohol can provide. There is no doubt that overconsumption of alcohol is unhealthy in the short and long term, and is not beneficial to our mental states. However, if you are able to find a form of alcohol that you can tolerate (and I do recognize that not everyone will), there is no reason for you not to indulge periodically if it makes you feel better. As with everything else in this section, it's all about moderation.

Some people may experience enough additional delays in emptying that the consumption of alcohol is not a positive experience. If you realize that this is the case for you, then you tried, and now you should steer clear!

GIVING THANKS

While this might seem like a throwaway concept initially, this is truly an important part of a management plan. Giving thanks for the good things that we do have in our lives forces us to focus on the positive and move our thoughts away from the negative. If I am thinking about how lucky I am to be able to take a hike through the woods, I'm probably not thinking about the pain in my stomach. If I am feeling grateful to be able to read so many books, I am probably not focusing on my constant regurgitation.

Letting the people in your life know that you are grateful for them is also a good practice to get into. Many of them are helping us to accommodate our needs and strange requests, and it is always good for them to know that we see and appreciate those efforts. On top of that, we really should be grateful! I have gone through points in my life where I didn't have anyone to fall back on, and it made those times when I had someone by my side all the more meaningful. I am sure many of you can express similar sentiments and experiences.

Self-Advocacy 23

"Opportunity is missed by most people because it is dressed in overalls and looks like work."

RALPH WALDO EMERSON

I would like to wrap up this book with a discussion on how to become your own best advocate. I cannot stress enough how important this is to guaranteeing your best health and finding the simplest path on your journey with gastroparesis. The information and skills that you have gained through this book are only as valuable as you make them. By becoming an advocate for your own health, you will not only be able to apply what you have learned here, but you will also establish for yourself a type of health independence. This independence can simplify your health management, grow your confidence, and improve your overall outlook and quality of life.

It may seem overwhelming or daunting at first to consider truly speaking up for yourself. I have already mentioned a number of times in my Personal Experience sections when I did not have the confidence or knowledge to speak up when I should have. However, after 15 years with this condition and my foray into actually working in the medical profession, I have one takeaway that trumps all others. I can tell you with concrete certainty that self-advocacy is the most precious tool that you have in improving your health. Unfortunately, it is not a commonly discussed or appreciated asset within our healthcare system, so it often goes unmentioned and underappreciated.

WHY IS SELF-ADVOCACY IMPORTANT?

You are the only constant in your care. For any symptom you experience, any doctor's office you go to, any visit to the emergency room, you are the only person that was present and involved in every single one of those events. You are the only consistent source of information regarding what you are experiencing. You are also the only consistent source of information for what you have tried and what you have not tried. Simply from the perspective of having all of the information on the table, you are the only person that can make sure this happens.

There may be some of you that have a committed health partner - be it a parent, spouse, or friend - that has also been there for each of these moments. Self-advocacy can be enhanced by a team approach for those of you that are lucky enough to have such a person in your life.

The condition that is being treated affects your body and yours alone. Your understanding for what is happening to your body or what needs to change is crucial to those changes being made. If your doctor wants you to try a medication or a new diet, you have to understand when and how to do these things or they won't work. You also have to understand why you are doing them, or you might give up too soon or ignore a side effect that you should not have ignored. If you don't ask clarifying questions and confirm that what you heard or think you heard is correct, you are the one that will make mistakes.

You are intimately familiar with your own personal concerns and considerations. If a specific diet or medication will not work for you because of something that it requires, you are the one that knows this. If you have already tried a specific medication and it caused a severe side effect, you are the one that knows this. If you simply cannot comply with what the doctor is asking you to do in regards to an exercise regimen because of a physical limitation, again, you are the one who knows this. Relaying this information to the doctor is crucial in order to find solutions that will actually work for you.

Your health matters more to you than to anyone else. And with a condition like gastroparesis, your heath is directly tied to your quality of life, which certainly matters more to you than to anyone else. A specific side effect or symptom might be very troublesome for you even though your doctor just sees it as a number on a sheet or your friends think you are overreacting. But you are the only one that can determine if it is pulling down your quality of life, and the only one that can advocate for a positive change.

Ultimately, self-advocacy is important because when it comes to your health and quality of life, you are the one who is impacted the most and also the one who knows the most.

None of these points are meant to be condescending or demeaning. Before I entered the medical profession, I had trouble realizing every single one of these considerations. We expect our doctors to remember what we tell them, or our medical charts to speak the truth. But the sad facts are that neither of those things happen. And if something seems like a valid consideration to us, it's probably a valid consideration. We just don't realize that we're the ones responsible for bringing it up because we have so often been taught not to.

WHAT IS STANDING IN THE WAY?

There are a number of barriers in our way to realizing when and why we should speak up and advocate for ourselves. These barriers have been taught to us throughout our lives and through societal norms. Here are some of the most commonly overlooked realities:

1. Doctors are not a separate class of beings. They are humans, too. They make mistakes. They make assumptions. And they are not always right.

2. Not all doctors are good listeners, and that is not something that should just be accepted as the status quo. Your doctor cannot properly care for you if he is not listening.

3. Not all doctors are good communicators, and that is also not something that should just be accepted as the status quo. You cannot "follow

the doctor's orders" if you don't understand them.

Whether or not we are aware of it, we all approach doctors as separate from us. We see them as more knowledgeable and more powerful, and we defer to their authority when we are sitting in their offices or hospitals. We take their words as fact and we do not question what we don't understand. There have actually been a number of psychological studies conducted that confirm this finding time and time again – as a society, we automatically defer to our physicians.

This leads me to the second set of barriers that must be knocked down – our many assumptions regarding doctors, our relationship to them, and our role in that relationship.

1. We assume that doctors only want to hear specific things and nothing more. Whether or not this is true, it is not appropriate. If a doctor is looking at you as "Gastroparesis Case #25", you need to remind him that you are a person with a life and past attached to you.

2. We assume that doctors do not want us to ask questions. While doctors may initially seem perturbed or frustrated by questions, the fact of the matter is that they want you to get better. They want their ideas to work, and in order for that to happen, they need you to understand how to make them work.

3. We assume that we have nothing valuable to add. The fact is, your doctor has many other patients and many other concerns. He can't always remember your entire medical history or something that you talked about at the last visit. You are the only true source of this information and thus you always have something valuable to add.

We also make many assumptions about our healthcare system as a whole that are unfortunately not true.

For instance, we expect our medical records to contain all of the information that is important. But they don't. Nor are they always available when we see a new doctor or end up at a different hospital.

Retail pharmacy companies do not even share information, so unless you fill all of your prescriptions with the same company, the pharmacist will not be able to safely evaluate all of the medications that you are taking.

HOW DO I BECOME A SELF-ADVOCATE?

The first step to becoming an active and useful participant in your own care is to beat down the preconceptions and roadblocks that are automatically standing in your way. Recognize that your doctor is not always right and that your doctor has obligations to you as a patient. Recognize that you have an obligation to yourself and something valuable to provide to your doctor. Any appointments should involve a two-sided discussion.

Steps to becoming a self-advocate:

1. Recognize that you need to be an active participant
2. Re-evaluate the members of your health team
3. Grow your confidence by building your knowledge
4. Develop ways to push yourself to participate

The next and very crucial step is to re-evaluate the members of your health team once you have climbed past those roadblocks. I can speak from experience in saying that your needs in a physician are different depending on where you are in your journey. When I was scared and sick, I needed a doctor that could explain things to me and that could stop to listen to my concerns. And it took me awhile to find him. As I became a stronger advocate for myself and developed a better grasp on my management plan, my needs began to change. Now that I have my condition under wraps and I understand what I need, I am fine with the doctor that hardly looks at me, checks the status of my pacemaker, asks if I need refills, and sends me on my way. We have a mutual understanding that very little is needed from each party.

So where are you at on your journey? Which doctor do you need? And now that you have begun to see your doctor as someone who is more on your level as opposed to a level above, do you feel that you are able to speak up and be heard? Does your doctor allow you to advocate for yourself? Does he stop to explain or listen when it is needed? You have an obligation to yourself to find a physician that is a better match for you. And this applies to your primary/general physician, your GI specialist, and any other specialists that you might need for other health issues that you experience.

The third step is developing a confidence in yourself and your knowledge that allows you to speak up when needed. This can be quite difficult at first. However, the information that you have learned from this book should help you to feel far more empowered as a patient and also far more confident in your abilities to understand what is happening to you and what is being suggested to you. Believe it or not, the knowledge that you have gained here will guide you in recognizing when something doesn't sound right for you, or in finding the right questions to ask. In fact, this knowledge will actually help you to realize where the holes are and which information is not clear to you – and those are always the right questions to ask.

When you are first pushing into the realm of self-advocacy, it might be helpful to use some special methods to make sure that you speak up for yourself. One great approach is to bring someone else with you to your appointments. Before you go in to the appointment, make sure that the other person knows exactly what you want to talk about, whether it is new ideas or new concerns that you have. This person can act as an accountability partner of sorts, ensuring that you have those specific discussions while you are there; that you don't lose your nerve or let yourself be shuttled out the door. And make sure that the other person has been given a free pass to speak up if something that they hear sounds off to them. The third person in the room is often more willing to speak up because they are not directly affected. If you cannot bring someone else with you, then bring a list and tell the doctor that you need to talk about each of the items on it before you leave. Whatever you need to do to get yourself going, do it!

Some tricks for overcoming an initial fear of speaking up can include:

- Bring someone with you
- Provide a list to the doctor
- Start small and work your way up to bigger issues
- Set doable goals for yourself
- Have an accountability partner hold you to following through, even if they are not actually present

THOUGHTS ON SELF-ADVOCACY

I want to close this section with some thoughts that I had while reading a book called The Laws of Medicine, by Dr. Siddhartha Mukherjee. This book was a culmination of his struggle to identify laws that apply to the field of medicine, which he openly admits must be laws of imperfection for an imperfect science. It was a shock to him to go from a school experience that involved compulsive naming and memorization of concrete facts to the lawless, uncertain world of clinical wisdom, which is imperfect and abstract.

Although he wrote the book and the laws to apply to physicians, when I read them they stood out to me as the laws that apply to the person with a chronic condition. For us, these laws are the exact reasons that we are such important pieces of our own care. To me, they are a call to self-advocacy.

STRONG INTUITION IS BETTER THAN WEAK TESTS

The intuition of the person with a chronic condition is incredibly strong. It takes time to establish; an intimate familiarity with the condition must first develop. But our intuitions should not be passed over or ignored, either by us or our medical providers. We are the most familiar with our bodies, we are the most familiar with our symptoms, and we are the most reliable source of information on what has and has not worked. If something strikes us as off or incorrect or concerning, we would be doing ourselves a disservice to not speak up. And this act of speaking up can be powerful in guiding the doctor to the right tests and the right treatments.

OUTLIERS CREATE LAWS

In medicine, a standard patient creates a rule, but it is the outlier that doesn't fit the rules that will eventually create the law. As people with gastroparesis, we often feel that we are the medical outliers. How long did it take for us to become diagnosed? How many doctors did we have to see to receive the right diagnosis? And how many doctors did we have to see to receive any adequate treatments?

As part of the medical system, we have an outlying diagnosis, one that is not well understood by the medical community, that presents dramatically differently between each person, and that is highly unpredictable in nature. Our laws have not yet been established, but as more of us seek treatment and advocate for our health, more information can be incorporated into the medical understanding of gastroparesis. If we commit to pushing forward for evidence and information that can improve our condition and the lives of others with gastroparesis, our outliers can be defined and bring us closer to that law.

HUMAN BIAS IS STRONG

Bias is easily identified in every human being, and just as easily so in those of us with chronic conditions. It is present in those administering medicine and those of us that are the subjects of that medicine. We develop our own thoughts and opinions as we endure our own experiences and excitements and disappointments.

We cement our thoughts on a topic based on our own successes and failures and we advocate and champion accordingly. But while this provides us a level of innate protection from making the same mistake twice or reliving a horrible experience, it is not always healthy or appropriate. It is our responsibility to recognize this bias within ourselves and guard against jumping to conclusions for others or giving advice that is not founded. We must also guard against being closed-minded to new options and treatments because of our existing biases regarding those options or even the person suggesting them.

The elimination of bias and pursuit of true understanding and valid information has been at the heart of this entire book. Armed with the tools and knowledge to create our own roadmaps, we can now answer the call to self-advocacy.

Personal Experience

The last time we were in my Personal Experience section I mentioned the point when I finally knew that I could live well. I want to introduce you to some of my strategies and my own personal management plan. However, because every person with gastroparesis is different, I will also make a point to mention the changes that I have tried and failed. Even though they failed for me, many of these changes have worked well for others.

I have already spoken about many of the components of my current management plan throughout the course of the book. This management plan could not have been developed without a dedicated evaluation of my medications, diet, and habits. I had to be willing to look at everything from an unbiased perspective and be willing to admit that what I was already doing was not cutting it and I needed to be open to ideas that might go against my preferences.

I no longer take any medications other than birth control (not oral!) and thyroid medication. This does not include the times that I need something in the moment. My go-to for pain relief is typically a gel-cap version of naproxen (Aleve). For sinus infections, I also turn to the gel-cap version of Advil Cold & Sinus. Traditionally, I was one of those people that never even thought to use medications for temporary issues. It took a long time for me to re-wire myself to the point where I now take something as soon as the symptoms appear (head cold, headache, joint pain, etc), knowing that it will take quite awhile to see the benefit.

I do have a standing anti-nausea prescription that I need to use 1-2 times per month. My baseline nausea that is ever-present is kept under control by managing my habits and using key food ingredients to help calm my stomach and my mind. For instance, the smell of ginger or mint is soothing to my stomach. However, I don't actually enjoy the strong flavors attached to either of those smells (go figure). So I will often grate ginger as a small component of a meal that I am making and I will sniff a mint product (candies, chocolates, teas) without eating it. I also have go-to 'plain' foods that I know that I can keep down when the going gets tough, such as plain brown rice, plain whole-wheat noodles, etc.

One thing that I have discovered over the years is that there are times when the action that seems the least logical is the one that I most need to consider. If I am experiencing particularly severe nausea and vomiting and believe that eating is my nemesis, sometimes eating is exactly what will calm my stomach. We often land ourselves in vicious cycles in which we are underfed, weak, and sick, which makes us more underfed, weaker, and sicker. In these times, if there is a specific food that my body is craving, I will eat it. Or I will try something bland that I know I have handled before, such as plain brown rice with melted mozzarella cheese. There was an exceptional amount of anxiety involved in my first taking this step, and I still have anxiety when these situations arise today. But I now recognize that desperate times call for desperate measures, and I trust that there is only 'up' from there.

While I have no way to stop my chronic regurgitation, it is not acidic. In fact, it became even less so when I stopped using my acid reducer that was originally prescribed by my doctor. I rely on Tums for those times when the food that is sitting in my stomach for hours on end becomes acidic and uncomfortable, and this occurs most often at night or in the morning (from the food that never emptied overnight).

My abdominal pain is sometimes difficult to tolerate, but I have not found that pain relievers are helpful during these times. Wearing clothing that is comfortable around the waist and using distraction techniques are two strategies that often do the trick much more effectively.

My nutrition is significantly improved from where I was ten years ago. I am able to prevent deficiencies simply by monitoring what I am getting in my diet on a weekly and monthly basis. But sometimes I am not as diligent as I should be and I make things more difficult for myself. For instance, while writing this book, I forgot to monitor my iron intake and became deficient again for the first time in seven years. I was definitely kicking myself for that one!

Portion control has become my best friend. I have found that I can even tolerate certain foods that do not go down very well if I consume them in very small quantities (even just one bite). The real benefit to this is the mental and emotional satisfaction of eating something I really love but cannot tolerate. But there are also times where consuming very small quantities has turned things around for me in an amazing way, such as in eating small bites of red meat off of other peoples' plates in order to maintain my iron levels.

Another discovery that was life-changing for me was the consistent consumption of a balance of sugar and protein. There is no clear way to tell anyone else how to do this - this took a lot of trial and error on my part. But whereas before I used to experience shaking and fainting episodes more than once a day, they have been reduced to occurring no more than once a week. This has been accomplished by always having a source of sugar on hand (and I mean always) and monitoring that I have adequate protein consumption in my meals. One great source of sugar for me is overripe fruit (such as soft pears). But I'll be completely honest - some days I suck on sugary candies to maintain my sugar balance. I'm not going to start lying to you now! It is what it is; we do what we have to do.

The big ticket concepts with a gastroparesis diet are 'low-fat' and 'low-fiber'. I need to take this opportunity to say that this generic guidance often does more harm than good. There are many different types of fiber, some of which are far more digestible than others. For instance, my overripe fruits are great sources of fiber. However, I avoid raw vegetables and salads like the plague, because they are impossible for my stomach to tolerate. If, however, I steam my veggies down to an unrecognizable pile of mush, some go down acceptably well. No one else that's around wants to eat them, but I've learned (with time) to love them in this form.

The 'low-fat' message has some merit in the sense that fats are harder for our stomachs to break down than carbohydrates and proteins. But proteins are also harder to break down than carbohydrates. So instead of looking at my food from the perspective of "low-fat", I see it as a world of ratios. Does this have a reasonable amount of protein and fat in it (for me)? Am I getting an adequate amount of protein in comparison to the fat content? Ok, perhaps I can try eating this item, cooked down, in small quantities, and go from there.

As I said, much of this is nothing more than trial and error, but it takes an openness to seeing things outside of the tiny boxes of 'low-fat, low-fiber' in order to do so. One person will tolerate different nutrients better or worse than someone else, and different manipulations will change this.

Speaking of manipulations, another topic worth addressing here is that of blending and juicing. To start, juicing is generally not a good idea because it removes the heart of the nutrients (the pulp) from the food. However, there are a lot of products out there now that retain nutrients, such as the Ninja. I personally do not handle blended or juiced items well. The density of the items cause my stomach to revolt, and I'll often end up curled up in pain. I have discovered that I am better able to tolerate certain items when they are cooked down as opposed to blended down. This is a different way of altering the actual food molecules. Cooking is a chemical manipulation, whereas blending is mechanical. If you are not tolerating one, it might be worth trying some options with the other.

Stress and time management are crucial factors in keeping my gastroparesis under control. But sometimes life gets difficult, whether professionally or personally, and hurdles cannot be avoided. In those times I turn to my comfort foods and my soda habit. While this used to be a source of shame for me, I am now able to recognize that maintaining comfortable places to retreat to is not a sign of weakness so much as an understanding of my limitations. These allow me to focus my energy where it is most needed, when it is most needed, so that I can tackle the obstacles and return to a better place.

A regular exercise routine factors into my stress management significantly. I guess calling it an exercise routine might be a bit of an exaggeration. It basically just involves a lot of walking. Consistent walking. Walking even when my stomach is hurting and my body is telling me to go sit on the couch and veg. At those times, I summon all of my willpower and I throw on a podcast or some music and I just go. Even if I don't get very far, I have never once regretted it.

I now only need to check in with my GI doctor once a year, during which time my neurostimulator is monitored. I check in with my primary physician twice a year and have my general health, thyroid, and nutrition monitored. I focus on the things that bring me joy, like reading, hiking, problem solving, playing instruments, and giving back. And I appreciate that I have the ability to focus on these things at all.

Afterword

The term "gastroparesis" is not one-size-fits-all. We are a community of unique people that each has our own personal version of this condition. For some of us it is quite severe. For others it is a manageable nuisance. Some people are otherwise healthy, while some are given a gastroparesis diagnosis on top of a whole slew of other chronic conditions - maybe even as a result of those other conditions. Regardless, as unintentional members of this community, we all have an opportunity to come together to provide support and guidance when we are struggling.

My website, www.YourGIJourney.com, is a space for people to find reliable, evidence-based information about the topics that collide with their GI conditions. It is meant to bridge the gap between you and your best health through the necessary, but often missing, information, knowledge, and guidance. In addition, it is continuously updated regarding advances in research, concepts making the rounds on the media circuit, and also new ideas and stories from those in similar situations to yours.

I cannot emphasize enough how important it is to be a self-advocate and to bring your management plan to its simplest state. Becoming informed and confident is not only necessary to receiving the best care, but also incredibly empowering. I did not become aware of its importance until I had endured significant struggles along my own journey. Self-advocacy and health simplification are concepts that I am very passionate about and believe are incredibly important to maintaining quality of life with a chronic condition.

I discuss these concepts in greater depth on the website. I also have a number of tools available that I developed specifically for the purpose of helping people to get on a path towards managing their health and simplifying their care. I believe that every person should have access to their best options, and that access should not be withheld or limited for any reason.

I could provide resources and generalized guidance until I'm blue in the face, and the truth is, it will help a lot of people to get answers to their questions. But in some situations, there is simply too much going on and is too much at play to figure this out on your own. Sometimes it just takes a guide with medical expertise and personal understanding to help out with the hardest parts. This website has provided me an opportunity to work directly with many people to figure out those hardest parts, piece by piece.

As you've seen throughout the book, my personal journey with gastroparesis has had its highs and lows. I will not lie about the fact that the lows predominated for quite some time. But I can say without hesitation that they are now few and far between and this has been the case for many years.

I spent a lot of time after my diagnosis thinking that I would find a way to 'overcome' or 'fix' what was happening to me. It took me years to come to terms with the fact that this was permanent and unfixable. Only after I had come to that realization was I truly ready to commit to helping myself and take charge of my own health.

While the road has not always been easy, I believe that it was absolutely worth travelling. I believe that the addition of severe gastroparesis to my life has had a tangible impact in shaping who I am. It has strengthened my character, increased my determination, and colored my empathy for others. The difficult days make me grateful for all of the good ones that I am able to have now, which has changed the way that I see my life and the world around me.

I wrote this book in an effort to allow others to learn from my mistakes. Perhaps the information provided here will prevent someone else from spinning their wheels the way that I did.

In addition, my training and role in the medical field ended up colliding with my personal experience to create an unintended but unique understanding for gastroparesis. I wanted as many people as possible to capitalize on this and jumpstart their own management.

I want to genuinely thank you for providing me with this opportunity to share my experiences and the tools for building a better quality of life.

If you filled out the survey when you started the book, you can complete your participation in the study with just one more minute of your time. And I won't leave you empty-handed afterwards! www.yourgijourney.com/s2

Acknowledgements

I have many people to thank for playing some part in making this book a reality. There are those that lovingly pushed me to believe that what I had to offer wasn't just of value, it was badass. I would like to thank each one of them for allowing me to see myself in a different light.

There are also the people that, with no kindness in their hearts whatsoever, forced me to step off of the cliff when I did not believe that I was ready. I have to thank each one of them for causing me to take a leap that I might not otherwise have taken.

My sincere gratitude must also be expressed to each person that read the words I have written and used them to live a better life - you've infused value into my work and are the only reason that it exists.

I could list names, but what would be the fun in that? Each person knows who they are. So without further ado, thank you for...

Being an infuriatingly persistent, loving, supportive, life-saving teammate.

Providing the spiritual duct tape of laminated bookmarks and punk rock.

Supporting Big Bird against the most critical of them all.

Being my everyman (and for all of the Chevy's chips), buddy.

Not pouring my blood, sweat, and tears down your drain (drvib Grg ro css).

Giving me life, my work ethic, and a frightening amount of determination.

Showing me that not everyone will open their eyes, and that not all of those who do will keep them open - those rare few are to be treasured indeed.

References

CHAPTER 2

Biesiekierski JR. Gluten causes gastrointestinal symptoms in subjects without celiac disease: a double-blind randomized placebo-controlled trial. Am J Gastroenterol. 2011 Mar;106(3):508-14

Clauson KA. Clinical Decision Support Tools: Analysis of Online Drug Information Databases. BMC Med Inform Decis Mak. 2007; 7: 7.

Egle JP. The Internet School of Medicine: Use of Electronic Resources by Medical Trainees and the Reliability of Those Resources. J Surg Educ. 2015 Mar-Apr;72(2):316-20. doi: 10.1016/j.jsurg.2014.08.005. Epub 2014 Dec 6.

CHAPTER 3

Bures J, Cyrany J, Kohoutova D, et al. Small intestinal bacterial overgrowth syndrome. World Journal of Gastroenterology : WJG. 2010;16(24):2978-2990. doi:10.3748/wjg.v16.i24.2978.

Ciorba MA. A Gastroenterologist's Guide to Probiotics. Clin Gastroenterol Hepatol 2012;10(9):960-968.

Dunn BE, Cohen H, Blaser MJ. Helicobacter Pylori. Clin Microbiol Rev. 1997 Oct;10(4):720-41.

Gorbach SL. Microbiology of the Gastrointestinal Tract. In: Baron S, editor. Medical Microbiology. 4th edition. Galveston (TX): University of Texas Medical Branch at Galveston; 1996. Chapter 95.

Nakamura RM. Laboratory tests for the evaluation of Helicobacter pylori infections. J Clin Lab Anal. 2001; 15(6):301-7.

Sachdev AH, Pimentel M. Gastrointestinal bacterial overgrowth: pathogenesis and clinical significance. Therapeutic Advances in Chronic Disease 2013; 4(5):223-231.

Thomas DW, Greer FR. Probiotics and Prebiotics in Pediatrics. Pediatrics 2010;126;1217.

CHAPTER 4

Rey E, Choung RS, Schleck CD, Zinsmeister AR, Talley NJ, Locke GR. Prevalence of Hidden Gastroparesis in the Community: The Gastroparesis "Iceberg." Journal of Neurogastroenterology and Motility. 2012;18(1):34-42.

CHAPTER 5

Aleksovski A, Dreu R, Gašperlin M, Planinšek O. Mini-tablets: a contemporary system for oral drug delivery in targeted patient groups. Expert Opin Drug Deliv. 2015 Jan;12(1):65-84

Heading RC, Nimmo J, Prescott LF, Tothill P. The dependence of paracetamol absorption on the rate of gastric emptying. Br J Pharmacol 1973;47:415-21.

Horowitz M, Su YC, Rayner CK, Jones KL. Gastroparesis: prevalence, clinical significance and treatment. Canadian Journal of Gastroenterology 2001 Dec;15(12):805-13.

Hunt JN. The regulation of gastric emptying. In: Modern Trends in Gastroenterology, ed. Avery Jones, F., pp163-176. Butterworth: London.

Sadiya A. Nutritional therapy for the management of diabetic gastroparesis: clinical review. Diabetes Metab Syndr Obes 2012;5:329-35.

Shepherd MF, Felt-Gunderson PA. Diarrhea associated with lorazepam solution in a tube-fed patient. Nutr Clin Pract. Jun 1996;11(3):117-120.

Smith TJ, Ritter JK, Poklis JL, et al. ABH gel is not absorbed from the skin of normal volunteers. J Pain Symptom Manage. 2012 May;43(5):961-6.

CHAPTER 6

Bennell J, Taylor C. A loss of social eating: the experience of individuals living with gastroparesis. Journal of Clinical Nursing 2012; 22: 2812-2821.

Berrill JW, Gallacher J, Hood K, et al. An observational study of cognitive function in patients with irritable bowel syndrome and inflammatory bowel disease. Neurogastroenterol Motil. 2013 Nov; 25(11):918-e704.

Bielefeldt K. Gastroparesis: Concepts, Controversies, and Challenges. Scientifica 2012.

Bielefeldt K, Raza S, Zickmund SL. Different faces of gastroparesis. World Journal of Gastroenterology 2009; 15(48): 6052-6060.

Bowen R. The Enteric Nervous System. Colorado State University website. Available at: http://arbl.cvmbs.colostate.edu/hbooks/pathphys/digestion/basics/gi_nervous.html. Accessed: August 24, 2016.

Camilleri M, Di Lorenzo C. The Brain-Gut Axis: From Basic Understanding to Treatment of Irritable Bowel Syndrome and Related Disorders. J Pediatr Gastroenterol Nutr 2012 April; 54(5):446-453.

Carabotti M, Scirocco A, Maselli MA, et al. The gut-brain axis: interactions between enteric microbiota, central and enteric nervous systems. Ann Gastroenterol. 2015 Apr-Jun; 28(2): 203-209.

Foster JA, McVey Neufeld KA. Gut-brain axis: how the microbiome influences anxiety and depression. Trends Neurosci. 2013 May; 36(5):305-12.

Frederico Azevedo et al., Equal numbers of neuronal and nonneuronal cells make the human brain an isometrically scaled-up primate brain. J. Comp. Neurol., 513: 532-541, 2009

Grundy D, Schemann M. Enteric Nervous System. Current Opinion in Gastroenterology 2007, 23:121-126

Hasler WL, Parkman HP, Wilson LA, et al. Psychological Dysfunction Is Associated With Symptom Severity but Not Disease Etiology or Degree of Gastric Retention in Patients With Gastroparesis. Am J Gastroenterol 2010; 105(11): 2357-2367.

Koloski NA, Jones M, Kalantar J, et al. The brain--gut pathway in functional gastrointestinal disorders is bidirectional: a 12-year prospective population-based study. Gut. 2012 Sep; 61(9):1284-90.

Koloski NA, Jones M, Kalantar J, et al. The brain-gut pathway in functional gastrointestinal disorders is bidirectional: a 12-year prospective population-based study. Gut 2012;61:1284-1290.

Konturek PC, Brzozowski T, Konturek SJ. Stress and the gut: pathophysiology, clinical consequences, diagnostic approach and treatment options. J Physiol Pharmacol. 2011 Dec;62(6):591-9.

Mikocka-Walus AA, Andrews JA, Bernstein CN, et al. Integrated Models of Care in Managing Inflammatory Bowel Disease: A Discussion. Inflamm Bowel Dis 2012;18:1582-1587.

Naseribafrouei A, Hestad K, Avershina E, et al. Correlation between the human fecal microbiota and depression. Neurogastroenterol Motil. 2014 Aug; 26(8):1155-62

Simrén M, Barbara G, Flint HJ, Spiegel BM, Spiller RC, Vanner S, Verdu EF, Whorwell PJ, Zoetendal EG, Rome Foundation Committee. Intestinal microbiota in functional bowel disorders: a Rome foundation report. Gut. 2013 Jan; 62(1):159-76.

CHAPTER 7

Aziz I, Hadjivassiliou M, Sanders DS. The Spectrum of Noncoeliac Gluten Sensitivity. Nat Rev Gastroenterol Hepatol. 2015 Sep;12(9):516-26.

Barrett JS, Gearry RB, Muir JG, et al. Dietary poorly absorbed, short-chain carbohydrates increase delivery of water and fermentable substrates to the proximal colon. Aliment Pharmacol Ther. 2010;31:874-882.

Chey WD, Kurlander J, Eswaran S. Irritable Bowel Syndrome: A Clinical Review. JAMA.2015;313(9):949-958.

Green PH, Lebwohl B, Greywoode R. Celiac Disease. J Allergy Clin Immunol. 2015 May;135(5):1099-106

Green PH, Krishnareddy S, Lebwohl B. Clinical Manifestations of Celiac Disease. Dig Dis 2015 Jun;60(6):1517-8

Lebowhl B, Leffler DA. Exploring the Strange New World of Non-Celiac Gluten Sensitivity. Clin Gastroenterol Hepatol, 2015 Sept;13(9):1613-5.

Magge S, Lembo A. Low-FODMAP Diet for Treatment of Irritable Bowel Syndrome. Gastroenterology & Hepatology. 2012;8(11):739-745.
Mozdiak Ella, O'Malley John, Arasaradnam Ramesh. Inflammatory bowel disease BMJ 2015; 351 :h4416

Rezaie A, Pimentel M, Rao SS. How to Test and Treat Small Intestinal Bacterial Overgrowth: an Evidence-Based Approach. Curr Gastroenterol Rep. 2016 Feb; 18(2):8.

Sachdev AH, Pimentel M. Gastrointestinal bacterial overgrowth: pathogenesis and clinical significance. Therapeutic Advances in Chronic Disease 2013; 4(5):223-231.

Tavakkoli A, Lewis SK, Tennyson CA, et al. Characteristics of Patients Who Avoid Wheat and/or Gluten in the Absence of Celiac Disease. Clin Gastroenterol Hepatol. 2014 Apr;12(4)632-5.

CHAPTER 8

FDA inspects supplement makers: T Tsouderos, "Dietary Supplements."

Geller AI, Shehab N, Weidle NJ. Emergency Department Visits for Adverse Events Related to Dietary Supplements. N Engl J Med 373;16

Gurley BJ, Gardner SF, Hubbard MA. Content versus label claims in ephedra-containing dietary supplements. Am J Health Syst Pharm 2000;57(10):963-9. Epub 2000/06/01. DOI

Hazell L, Shkir SAW. Under-reporting of adverse drug reactions: a systematic review. Drug Safety 2006; 29(5):385-96.

Kutz GD. Herbal Dietary Supplements: Examples of Deceptive or Questionable Marketing Practices and Potentially Dangerous Advice. 1 ed.

LeBlanc ES, Perrin N, Johnson JD, Jr., Ballatore A, Hillier T. Over-the-counter and compounded vitamin D: is potency what we expect? JAMA Intern Med 2013;173(7):585-6.

Navarro, V., Khan, I., Björnsson, E., Seeff, L. B., Serrano, J. and Hoofnagle, J. H. (2016), Liver Injury from Herbal and Dietary Supplements. Hepatology. Accepted Author Manuscript.

Newmaster SG, Grguric M, Shanmughanandhan D, Ramalingam S, Ragupathy S. DNA barcoding detects contamination and substitution in North American herbal products. BMC Med 2013;11:222.

Parasrampuria J, Schwartz K, Petesch R. Quality control of dehydroepi-androsterone dietary supplement products. JAMA 1998;280(18):1565. Epub 1998/11/20.

The Drug Development Process Step 3: Clinical Research. U.S. Food and Drug Administration/Center fr Drug Evaluation and Research. Available at: http://www.fda.gov/ForPatients/Approvals/Drugs/ucm405622.htm. Accessed on: Sept 12, 2016.

U. S. Food and Drug Administration/Center for Drug Evaluation and Research. (2009). FDA Advises Consumers Not To Use Certain Zicam Cold Remedies Intranasal Zinc Product Linked to Loss of Sense of Smell: FDA public health advisory. Washington, DC.

U.S. Food and Drug Administration/Center for Drug Evaluation and Research. Final rule declaring dietary supplements containing ephedrine alkaloids adulterated because they present an unreasonable risk. Federal Register;69(28):6787-854.

Webb G. "fX": chemically adulterated product does not contain kava. Herbalgram;39:9.

Zivin JA. Understanding Clinical Trials. Scientific American, April 2000

CHAPTER 9

Coffman B. A Cautionary Tale: The Risks of Unproven Antimalarials. Centers for Disease Control and Prevention website. Available at: https://www.cdc.gov/malaria/stories/homeopathic_drugs.html. Accessed: Sept 12, 2016.

Ernst, E. 'A systematic review of systematic reviews of homeopathy' Br J Clin Pharmacol 2002; 54:577-82.

Ernst, E. 'Acupuncture – a critical analysis', J Intern Med 2006; 259:125-37.

E. Ernst, "Deaths after acupuncture: A systematic Review," International Journal of Risk and Safety in Medicine 22 (2010):131-36.
Natural Standard Herb & Supplement Guide: An Evidence-Based Reference, 1e 1st Edition

Sample, Ian. "Dozens Killed by Incorrectly Placed Acupuncture Needles," The Guardian, October 18,2010.

Shang, A., et al. 'Are the clinical effects of homeopathy placebo effects? Compartive study of placebo-controlled trials of homeopathy and allopathy'. Lancet 2005; 366:726-32.

Tony Carllson, Liv Bergqvist, Urban Hellgren. Homeopathic Resistant Malaria. Journal of Travel Medicine Mar 1996, 3 (1) 62

U. S. Food and Drug Administration/Center for Drug Evaluation and Research. (2010). Hyland's Teething Tablets: Recall - Risk of Harm to Children: FDA public health advisory. Washington, DC.

U. S. Food and Drug Administration/Center for Drug Evaluation and Research. (2016). FDA warns against the use of homeopathic teething tablets and gels: FDA public health advisory. Washington, DC.

U. S. Food and Drug Administration/Center for Drug Evaluation and Research (2014). Terra-Medica Issues Voluntary Nationwide Recall of Specified Lots of Pleo Homeopathic Drug Products Due to the Potential for Undeclared Penicillin: FDA public health advisory. Washington, DC.

Woo Patrick C Y, Lin Ada W C, Lau Susanna K P, Yuen Kwok-Yung. Acupuncture transmitted infections BMJ 2010; 340:c1268.

CHAPTER 10

Atwell LL, Hsu A, Wong CP, et al. Absorption and chemopreventive targets of sulforaphane in humans following consumption of broccoli sprouts or a myrosinase-treated broccoli sprout extract. Molecular nutrition & food research. 2015;59(3):424-433.

Bjelakovic G, Gluud LL, Nikolova D, et al. Vitamin D supplementation for prevention of mortality in adults. Cochrane Database Syst Rev. 2014 Jan 10;1:CD007470.

Dietary Reference Intakes (DRIs): Elements. National Academies of Nutrition website. Available at: http://nationalacademies.org/hmd/~/media/Files/Activity%20Files/Nutrition/DRIs/New%20Material/6_%20Elements%20Summary.pdf

Dietary Reference Intakes (DRIs): Vitamins. National Academies of Nutrition website. Available at: http://nationalacademies.org/hmd/~/media/Files/ Activity%20Files/Nutrition/DRIs/New%20Material/7_%20Nutrients%20 Summary.pdf

Holick MF. Vitamin D deficiency. N Engl J Med 2007;357:266-81

Holick MF. Vitamin D: the underappreciated D-lightful hormone that is important for skeletal and cellular health. Curr Opin Endocrinol Diabetes 2002;9:87-98.

Nutrient bioavailability – getting the most out of food. European Food Information Council website. Available at: http://www.eufic.org/article/ en/artid/Nutrient-bioavailability-food/

CHAPTER 11

McIntyre CM, Monk HM. Medication absorption considerations in patients with postpyloric enteral feeding tubes. Am J Hosp Pharm. 2014 Apr (71):549-56.

Niv E, Fireman Z, Vaisman N. Post-pyloric feeding. World Journal of Gastroenterology : WJG. 2009;15(11):1281-1288. doi:10.3748/wjg.15.1281.

CHAPTER 12

Brogden RN, Carmine AA, Heel RC, et al. Domperidone. A review of its pharmacological activity, pharmacokinetics, and therapeutic efficacy in the symptomatic treatment of chronic dyspepsia and as an antiemetic. Drugs 1982; 24(5):360-400.

Domperidone Maleate – Association with Serious Abnormal Heart Rhythms and Sudden Death (Cardiac Arrest). Accessed at: http://www.healthycana-dians.gc.ca/recall-alert-rappel-avis/hc-sc/2012/14118a-eng.php. March 7, 2012.

Domperidone [package insert]. Australia: Janssen-CILAG Pty Ltd, 2012.

Gold Standard, Inc. Cisapride. Clinical Pharmacology [database online]. Available at:http://www.clinicalpharmacology.com. Accessed: September 5, 2016.

Gold Standard, Inc. Erythromycin. Clinical Pharmacology [database online]. Available at: http://www.clinicalpharmacology.com. Accessed: September 5, 2016.

Gold Standard, Inc. Metoclopramide. Clinical Pharmacology [database online]. Available at: http://www.clinicalpharmacology.com. Accessed: September 5, 2016.

Jones MP. Access Options for Withdrawn Motility-Modifying Agents. The American Journal of Gastroenterology 2002; 97(9):2184-88.

Mohammed F. Withdrawal of cisapride. BMJ 2001;323:1354

Parkman HP, Mishra A, Jacobs M, et al. Clinical Response and Side Effects of Metoclopramide. Journal of Clinical Gastroenterology 2012; 46:494-503.

Sanger, G. J. (2014), Ghrelin and motilin receptor agonists: time to introduce bias into drug design. Neurogastroenterol. Motil., 26: 149–155.

CHAPTER 13

Abell TL, Johnson WD, Kedar A, et al. A double-masked, randomized, placebo-controlled trial of temporary endoscopic mucosal gastric electrical stimulation for gastroparesis. Gastrointest Endosc. 2011; 74:496–503.

Abell T, McCallum R, Hocking M, et al. Gastric electrical stimulation for medically refractory gastroparesis. Gastroenterology. 2003; 125:421–428.

Arts J, Holvoet L, Caenepeel P, et al. Clinical trial: a randomized-controlled crossover study of intrapyloric injection of botulinum toxin in gastroparesis. Aliment Pharmacol Ther. 2007 Nov 1;26(9):1251-8.

Bai Y, Xu MJ, Yang X, et al. A systematic review on intrapyloric botulinum toxin injection for gastroparesis. Digestion. 2010; 81(1):27-34.

Camilleri M, Parkman HP, Shafi MA, et al. Clinical Guideline: Management of Gastroparesis. Am J Gastroenterol. 2013 January; 108(1):18-38.

Chu H, Lin Z, Zhong L, et al. A meta-analysis: the treatment of high-frequency gastric electrical stimulation for gastroparesis. J Gastroenterol Hepatol. 2012; 27:1017-1026.

Friedenberg FK, Palit A, Parkman HP. Botulinum toxin A for treatment of delayed gastric emptying. Am J Gastroenterol. 2008 Feb; 103(2):416-23.

McCallum R, Snape WJ Jr. Wo JM, et al. Enterra® gastric electrical stimulation for idiopathic gastroparesis: results from a multicenter randomized study. Gastroenterology. 2010; 138:1065.

O'Grady G, Egbuji JU, Du P, et al. High-frequency gastric electrical stimulation for the treatment of gastroparesis: a meta-analysis. World J Surg. 2009; 33:1693–1701.

CHAPTER 14

Chubineh S, Birk J. Proton pump inhibitors: the good, the bad, and the unwanted. South Med J 2012 Nov; 105(11):613-18.

Forgacs I, Loganayagam A. Overprescribing proton pump inhibitors is expensive and not evidence-based. British Medical Journal 2008;336:2-3.

Gold Standard, Inc. Ranitidine. Clinical Pharmacology [database online]. Available at: http://www.clinicalpharmacology.com. Accessed: September 6, 2016.

Gold Standard, Inc. Famotidine. Clinical Pharmacology [database online]. Available at: http://www.clinicalpharmacology.com. Accessed: September 6, 2016.

Gold Standard, Inc. Calcium carbonate. Clinical Pharmacology [database online]. Available at: http://www.clinicalpharmacology.com. Accessed: September 6, 2016.

Gold Standard, Inc. Magnesium Hydroxide. Clinical Pharmacology [database online]. Available at: http://www.clinicalpharmacology.com. Accessed: September 6, 2016.

Hershcovici T, Fass R. Pharmacological management of GERD: Where does it stand now? Trends Pharmacol Sci 2011 Apr; 32(4):258-64.

Hess MW, Hoenderop JG, Bindels RJ, Drenth JP. Systematic review: hypomagnesaemia induced by proton pump inhibition. Aliment Pharmacol Ther 2012 Sep; 36(5):405-13.

Katz MH. Failing the Acid Test: Benefits of proton pump inhibitors may not justify the risks for many users. Arch Intern Med 2010 May; 170(9):747-478.

Madanick RD. Proton Pump Inhibitor Side Effects and Drug Interactions: Much Ado About Nothing? Cleveland Clinic Journal of Medicine 2011 Jan; 78(1):39-49.

Vine L, Philpott R, Fortun P. Proton pump inhibitors: How to withdraw treatment. Prescriber 2012 Sep; 23(18):12-16.

CHAPTER 15

Gold Standard, Inc. Polyethylene Glycol. Clinical Pharmacology [database online]. Available at: http://www.clinicalpharmacology.com. Accessed: September 6, 2016.

Gold Standard, Inc. Bisacodyl. Clinical Pharmacology [database online]. Available at: http://www.clinicalpharmacology.com. Accessed: September 6, 2016.

Gold Standard, Inc. Sennosides. Clinical Pharmacology [database online]. Available at: http://www.clinicalpharmacology.com. Accessed: September 6, 2016.

Gold Standard, Inc. Magnesium hydroxide. Clinical Pharmacology [database online]. Available at: http://www.clinicalpharmacology.com. Accessed: September 6, 2016.

Gold Standard, Inc. Docusate. Clinical Pharmacology [database online]. Available at: http://www.clinicalpharmacology.com. Accessed: September 6, 2016.

Gold Standard, Inc. Magnesium Citrate. Clinical Pharmacology [database online]. Available at: http://www.clinicalpharmacology.com. Accessed: September 6, 2016.

Gold Standard, Inc. Mineral Oil. Clinical Pharmacology [database online]. Available at: http://www.clinicalpharmacology.com. Accessed: September 6, 2016.

Gold Standard, Inc. Sodium Phosphate Monobasic Monohydrate; Sodium Phosphate Dibasic Anhydrous. Clinical Pharmacology [database online]. Available at: http://www.clinicalpharmacology.com. Accessed: September 6, 2016.

CHAPTER 16

Gold Standard, Inc. Diphenhydramine. Clinical Pharmacology [database online]. Available at: http://www.clinicalpharmacology.com. Accessed: September 6, 2016.

Gold Standard, Inc. Meclizine. Clinical Pharmacology [database online]. Available at: http://www.clinicalpharmacology.com. Accessed: September 6, 2016.

Gold Standard, Inc. Promethazine. Clinical Pharmacology [database online]. Available at: http://www.clinicalpharmacology.com. Accessed: September 6, 2016.

Gold Standard, Inc. Ondansetron. Clinical Pharmacology [database online]. Available at: http://www.clinicalpharmacology.com. Accessed: September 6, 2016.

Gold Standard, Inc. Granisetron. Clinical Pharmacology [database online]. Available at: http://www.clinicalpharmacology.com. Accessed: September 6, 2016.

Gold Standard, Inc. Trimethobenzamide. Clinical Pharmacology [database online]. Available at: http://www.clinicalpharmacology.com. Accessed: September 6, 2016.

Natural Medicines Comprehensive Database. Stockton, CA: Therapeutic Research Faculty; 2013.http://naturaldatabase.therapeuticresearch.com/. Accessed September 6, 2016.

CHAPTER 17

Clarke G, Cryan JF, Dinan TG, Quigley EM. Review article: Probiotics for the treatment of irritable bowel syndrome – focus on lactic acid bacteria. Aliment Pharmacol Ther 2012; 35:403-413.

George, N.S., Sankineni, A. & Parkman, H.P. Dig Dis Sci (2014) 59: 645.

Gold Standard, Inc. Rifaximin. Clinical Pharmacology [database online]. Available at: http://www.clinicalpharmacology.com. Accessed: September 13, 2016.

Gold Standard, Inc. Neomycin. Clinical Pharmacology [database online]. Available at: http://www.clinicalpharmacology.com. Accessed: September 13, 2016.

Hempel S, Newberry S, Ruelaz A, et al. Safety of Probiotics to Reduce Risk and Prevent or Treat Disease. Evidence Report/Technology Assessment No. 200. (Prepared by the Southern California Evidence-based Practice Center under Contract No. 290-2007-10062-I.) AHRQ Publication No. 11-E007. Rockville, MD: Agency for Healthcare Research and Quality. April 2011. Available at: www.ahrq.gov/clinic/tp/probiotictp.htm

Meijer BJ, Dieleman LA. Probiotics in the Treatment of Human Inflammatory Bowel Diseases. J Clin Gastroenterol 2011;45:S139–S144.

Rezaie, A., Pimentel, M. & Rao, S.S. How to Test and Treat Small Intestinal Bacterial Overgrowth: an Evidence-Based Approach. Curr Gastroenterol Rep (2016) 18: 8

Ringel Y, Ringel-Kulka T. The Rationale and Clinical Effectiveness of Probiotics in Irritable Bowel Syndrome. J Clin Gastroenterol 2011;45:S145–S148.

Ringel Y, Quigley EMM, Lin HC. Using Probiotics in GI Disorders. Am J Gastroenterol Suppl 2012; 1:34–40.

Shah SC, Day LW, Somsouk M, and Sewell JL. Meta-analysis: antibiotic therapy for small intestinal bacterial overgrowth. Aliment Pharmacol Ther 2013; 38(8):1–10.

Szajewska H, Koldziej M. Systematic review with meta-analysis: Lactobacillus rhamnosus GG in the prevention of antibiotic-associated diarrhoea in children and adults. Aliment Pharmacol Ther 2015 Nov;42(10):1149–57.

CHAPTER 18

Gold Standard, Inc. Mirtazapine. Clinical Pharmacology [database online]. Available at: http://www.clinicalpharmacology.com. Accessed: September 9, 2016.

Gold Standard, Inc. Buspirone. Clinical Pharmacology [database online]. Available at: http://www.clinicalpharmacology.com. Accessed: September 9, 2016.

Grover M, Drossman DA. Psychopharmacologic and Behavioral Treatments for Functional Gastrointestinal Disorders. Gastrointest Endoscopy Clin N Am 19 (2009) 151-170.

Parkman HP, Camilleri M, Farrugia G, et al. Gastroparesis and Functional Dyspepsia: Excerpts from the AGA/ANMS Meeting. Neurogastroenterol Motil 2010; 22(2): 113-133.

Talley NJ, Locke GR, Herrick LM, et al. Functional Dyspepsia Treatment Trial: A Double-blind, Randomized, Placebo-controlled Trial of Antidepressants in Functional Dyspepsia, Evaluating Symptoms, Psychopathology, Pathophysiology, and Pharmacogenetics. Contemporary Clinical Trials 2012; 33: 523-533

Thorkelson G, Bielefeldt K, Szigethy E. Empirically Supported Use of Psychiatric Medications in Adolescents and Adults with IBD. Inflamm Bowel Dis 2016;22:1509-1522.

CHAPTER 19

Gold Standard, Inc. Melatonin. Clinical Pharmacology [database online]. Available at: http://www.clinicalpharmacology.com. Accessed: September 9, 2016.

Gold Standard, Inc. Zolpidem. Clinical Pharmacology [database online]. Available at: http://www.clinicalpharmacology.com. Accessed: September 9, 2016.

Gold Standard, Inc. Eszopiclone. Clinical Pharmacology [database online]. Available at: http://www.clinicalpharmacology.com. Accessed: September 9, 2016.

Gold Standard, Inc. Ramelteon. Clinical Pharmacology [database online]. Available at: http://www.clinicalpharmacology.com. Accessed: September 9, 2016.

Gold Standard, Inc. Tasimelteon. Clinical Pharmacology [database online]. Available at: http://www.clinicalpharmacology.com. Accessed: September 9, 2016.

Gold Standard, Inc. Zaleplon. Clinical Pharmacology [database online]. Available at: http://www.clinicalpharmacology.com. Accessed: September 9, 2016.

CHAPTER 20

Caballero-Plasencia AM, Valenzuela-Barranco M, Martín-Ruiz JL, et al. Are there changes in gastric emptying during the menstrual cycle? Scand J Gastroenterol. 1999 Aug;34(8):772-6.

Espey E, Ogburn T. Long-Acting Reversible Contraceptives - Intrauterine Devices and the Contraceptive Implant. Obstet Gynecol 2011;117:705-19.

Gold Standard, Inc. Medroxyprogesterone. Clinical Pharmacology [database online]. Available at: http://www.clinicalpharmacology.com. Accessed: September 9, 2016.

Gold Standard, Inc. Norelgestromin - ethinyl estradiol. Clinical Pharmacology [database online]. Available at: http://www.clinicalpharmacology.com. Accessed: September 9, 2016.

Roumen FJ, Mishell DR. The contraceptive vaginal ring, NuvaRing(®), a decade after its introduction. Eur J Contracept Reprod Health Care. 2012 Dec; 17(6):415-27.

Verrengia, M., Sachdeva, P., Gaughan, J., Fisher, R. S. and Parkman, H. P. (2011), Variation of symptoms during the menstrual cycle in female patients with gastroparesis. Neurogastroenterology & Motility, 23: 625–e254.

CHAPTER 21

Camilleri M, Parkman HP, Shafi MA, et al. Clinical Guideline: Management of Gastroparesis. Am J Gastroenterol. 2013 January; 108(1):18-38.

Living with Diabetes Complications: Gastroparesis. American Diabetes Association website. Available at: http://www.diabetes.org/living-with-diabetes/complications/gastroparesis.html?referrer=https://www.google.com/

Index

About the Author

Chelsey M McIntyre, PHARMD is a clinical pharmacist with chronic gastroparesis whose appetite for learning never went away. She has a love for reading and gets as excited about research and science as she does for her next adventure in the Columbia River Gorge.

She is the founder of Your GI Journey, where she has committed to making accesible to everyone the tools and information needed to improve health with chronic GI diagnoses.

So sad to have reached the end? Visit the website for even more learning!

www.YourGIJourney.com

Made in the USA
Columbia, SC
25 February 2021